'This is a fascinating collection of Frigga Haug's essays on topics ranging from feminist theory and methodology to the relationship between productive and reproductive labor to post-capitalist utopian imaginaries. Expertly bookended by the editors' incisive introduction and a wide-ranging interview with Haug, these essays provide Anglophone readers with an essential introduction to her ground-breaking body of work. Essential reading for anyone interested in contemporary critical theory.'

Amy Allen, *The Pennsylvania State University, USA*

Selected Writings of Frigga Haug on Experience, Labour, and Critique

This book offers a compelling introduction to the groundbreaking work of one of Germany's most influential feminist and Marxist thinkers, Frigga Haug. For over five decades, Haug's writings have shaped critical debates on gender, subjectivity, and social transformation, yet much of her work has remained inaccessible to English-speaking audiences until now.

This collection brings together a selection of her most thought-provoking essays, making her profound insights available to a wider readership. At the core of Haug's intellectual and political practice is a radical insistence on the interplay between subjective experience and structural oppression. Her essays explore how the oppressed are often complicit in reproducing their own subjugation, while also offering a vision of transformation rooted in everyday life. Through her nuanced engagement with philosophy, sociology, psychoanalysis, and Marxism, Haug challenges readers to see theory and practice as inseparable, inviting them to rethink feminist politics and social change in the context of contemporary struggles.

This volume is an essential resource for scholars, students, and critical thinkers in fields such as feminism, Marxism, psychoanalysis, philosophy, and social theory, and provides a rich and transformative perspective on the challenges of our time.

Jeta Mulaj is Assistant Professor of Philosophy at Toronto Metropolitan University, Canada. Her research focuses on political philosophy, feminist philosophy, critical theory, Marxism, and psychoanalysis. She is the co-founder and executive director of the Balkan Society for Theory and Practice and a research associate for the Society for Women of Ideas.

Alexandra Colligs is a postdoctoral researcher at the University of Kassel, Germany. Her research focuses are social philosophy, critical theory, feminist theory, aesthetics, and philosophy of mind. She is the author of *Identität und Befreiung* (Campus 2021) and co-editor of *Kritische Theorie und Feminismus* [Critical Theory and Feminism] (Suhrkamp 2022).

Cindy Zeiher (translator) is a Lacanian psychoanalyst in training, translator, and senior lecturer at the University of Canterbury, New Zealand, where she teaches modernist and postmodernist critical theories in the human services program. Her writings explore Freudian-Lacanian interventions and interpretations relating to the contemporary nexus of subjectivity, ontology, and desire.

Philosophy and Psychoanalysis Book Series
Jon Mills
Series Editor

Philosophy and Psychoanalysis is dedicated to current developments and cutting-edge research in the philosophical sciences, phenomenology, hermeneutics, existentialism, logic, semiotics, cultural studies, social criticism, and the humanities that engage and enrich psychoanalytic thought through philosophical rigor. With the philosophical turn in psychoanalysis comes a new era of theoretical research that revisits past paradigms while invigorating new approaches to theoretical, historical, contemporary, and applied psychoanalysis. No subject or discipline is immune from psychoanalytic reflection within a philosophical context including psychology, sociology, anthropology, politics, the arts, religion, science, culture, physics, and the nature of morality. Philosophical approaches to psychoanalysis may stimulate new areas of knowledge that have conceptual and applied value beyond the consulting room reflective of greater society at large. In the spirit of pluralism, *Philosophy and Psychoanalysis* is open to any theoretical school in philosophy and psychoanalysis that offers novel, scholarly, and important insights in the way we come to understand our world.

Titles in this series:

A Psycho-Political Analysis of Netanyahu's Israel: The Israeli Anxiety
Itzhak Benyamini

A Philosophical Framework for Psychotherapy Integration: Psychoanalysis Meets Otherness
Yael Peri Herzovich and Aner Govrin

Selected Writings of Frigga Haug on Experience, Labour, and Critique
Jeta Mulaj and Alexandra Colligs

Please visit our website to find out more about this series: www.routledge.com/Philosophy-and-Psychoanalysis/book-series/PHILPSY

Selected Writings of Frigga Haug on Experience, Labour, and Critique

Edited by Jeta Mulaj and Alexandra Colligs

Translated by Cindy Zeiher, in collaboration with Alexandra Colligs and Jeta Mulaj

Routledge
Taylor & Francis Group
LONDON AND NEW YORK

Cover Design Credit: Threads of Domination © Kathryna Cuizon

First published in English 2027
by Routledge
4 Park Square, Milton Park, Abingdon, Oxon OX14 4RN

and by Routledge
605 Third Avenue, New York, NY 10158

Routledge is an imprint of the Taylor & Francis Group, an informa business

Translated by Cindy Zeiher, in collaboration with Alexandra Colligs and Jeta Mulaj.

British Library Cataloguing-in-Publication Data
A catalogue record for this book is available from the British Library

ISBN: 978-1-032-76803-8 (hbk)
ISBN: 978-1-032-76801-4 (pbk)
ISBN: 978-1-003-48014-3 (ebk)

DOI: 10.4324/9781003480143

Typeset in Times New Roman
by codeMantra

Contents

Editors' Preface

Alexandra Colligs and Jeta Mulaj

This volume brings together a selection of essays, articles, and speeches by Frigga Haug, one of the most influential feminist and Marxist thinkers in Germany. Over more than five decades, Haug's work has profoundly shaped debates on gender, subjectivity, and social transformation. Yet, only a small portion of her writings has so far been available in English. This collection seeks to make Haug's thought accessible to a wider readership and to underscore the continuing relevance of her projects for contemporary feminist theory, Marxism, and critical theory.

At the heart of Haug's intellectual and political practice, as well as her activism, lies an insistence on the weight of subjective experience and the critical insight that the oppressed are themselves implicated in reproducing their own subjection. Following this insight, she developed a new feminist methodology called "memory work" as a tool to analyze the intricate relationship between subjective experience and objective social structures. Haug's ideas—at once theoretical, political, and deeply self-reflexive—remain indispensable for understanding both the enduring mechanisms of domination and the possibilities for emancipation that arise within them.

Born in Mülheim, Germany, in 1937, Haug devoted her life equally to intellectual inquiry and academic work and to political activism and organizing. Until 2001, she served as Professor of Sociology at the University for Economics and Politics in Hamburg, and she has held visiting professorships in Klagenfurt, Innsbruck, Copenhagen (Denmark), Sydney (Australia), Toronto (Canada), and Durham (USA). She is the co-editor of the journal *Das Argument* and the *Historisch-Kritisches Wörterbuch des Marxismus* (Historical-Critical Dictionary of Marxism), an ongoing multi-volume collective project. She also founded the feminist crime series *Ariadne* and is the author of two crime novels. Among Haug's most important books—of which only a few can be mentioned here—are *Sexualisierung der Körper* [Sexualization of Bodies] (1991), *Beyond Female Masochism: Memory Work and Politics* (1992), *Frauen-Politiken* [Women's Politics] (1996), *Erinnerungsarbeit* [Memory Work] (2001), *Lernverhältnisse: Selbstbewegungen und Selbstblockierungen* [Learning Relations: Self-Movements and Self-Blockades] (2003), *Rosa Luxemburg und die Kunst der Politik*

[Rosa Luxemburg and the Art of Politics] (2004), *Die Vier-in-einem-Perspektive: Politik von Frauen für eine neue Linke* [The Four-in-One Perspective: Women's Politics for a New Left] (2008), and *Der im Gehen erkundete Weg* [The Path Explored While Walking] (2015).

In bringing some of Haug's writings together, this volume invites readers to trace the unfolding of a sustained political and intellectual project—an effort to think transformation through everyday life, to encounter theory and practice as mutually informing endeavors, and to insist that the collective and the personal, the subjective and the objective, are never entirely separate terrains. In revisiting Haug's work, this volume seeks not only to honor a remarkable body of thought but also to make available a perspective from which to rethink feminist politics today.

For this volume, we are deeply grateful to Frigga, who welcomed us warmly and actively participated in the selection of the texts included here. This project would not have been possible without her guidance and enthusiasm. We also extend our thanks to Wolfgang Fritz Haug, whose care and hospitality sustained us during our time with Frigga and who generously engaged in long conversations about their shared projects and life together. Special gratitude goes to Cindy Zeiher, who shares our enthusiasm for Frigga's work. Her extraordinary translations were crucial to bringing this volume into fruition. We are also indebted to Arianna Bullett, who meticulously transcribed the English portions of our extensive interview, and to Luca Di Maio, whose diligent assistance with references and citations was invaluable.

We hope this collection of essays will spark renewed interest in the work of Frigga Haug, whose profound contributions to Marxism and feminism are sure to advance academic debates and activism in the Anglophone context.

Untying the Domination Knot: Editors' Introduction

Alexandra Colligs and Jeta Mulaj

Our first real encounter with Frigga Haug was disorienting. We had flown to La Palma and, in a rented car, wound our way through the island's impossibly narrow, twisting roads in the dark, the sea hidden just beyond the edge, on our way to meet her for the interview that would eventually give rise to this volume. Frigga and her husband Wolf welcomed us with a warmth that dispelled the fatigue of the journey. Once we settled into the Don Quixote guesthouse, we sat smoking on the terrace, enjoying the silence broken only by the waves and the birds. The sun was sinking behind the strip of beach to which, as we were later told, Frigga and Wolf had once fled from a fire, and where, she added in passing, she and her feminist study groups used to go swimming between their intense discussions.

In the days that followed, our work absorbed us so completely that we never once made it to the beach ourselves. Between long conversations we wandered through their vast grounds where they cultivated all kinds of fruit and vegetables, the basis of every meal we shared. We even acquired a few practical insights into agricultural science—what could flourish in that peculiar island climate: vines heavy with tomatoes, lemons swelling in the sun, fruits whose flavors were entirely new to us. By the end of our stay, we had even learned how to harvest potatoes.

For our initial conversation with Frigga, we had done what is customary in academic settings: studied her work closely and prepared a list of questions that carefully traced its conceptual threads. To our surprise, Frigga seemed not only unimpressed but at times genuinely puzzled, perhaps even irritated, by our theoretical elaborations and carefully planned inquiries. What she found missing, she told us, was what she called "our standpoint." Having passed through an academic training that dismissed subjective experience and individual perspective as irrelevant, or at best anecdotal, to theoretical inquiry, we were, in turn, bewildered. Yet, in the days that followed, as our conversations unfolded and Frigga's insistence on "our standpoint" persisted with a stubborn rigor, we came to understand and experience that her theoretical work is rooted in a specific practice of relating to others—one that refuses to allow the so-called private realm to remain at rest, instead insisting that it be drawn into theory and politics. As in her work, so in our conversations, that which has been historically deemed unworthy of philosophical reflection—from the reproduction of human material existence to the compulsory labour of breastfeeding—revealed itself as the sediment of socio-historical processes that places the highest demands on theory.

Much of Frigga's work has been preoccupied with the oppressed, especially women long deprived of the right to speak for themselves. Their particular experiences have been tucked behind, not even subsumed within, the universal, male ones, such that whenever they emerged at all, they did so only as trivialities, as the idle chatter of those who "know nothing of life." In this context, Frigga Haug's writings enact a Copernican reversal: the lives of women, their labour, understandings, fears, anxieties, and daily concerns become the center, the hidden axis around which everything turns. To speak for oneself as a way of testifying to lived experience sheds its triviality and reveals the ideological falsity of a society whose alleged universality rests on domination. Indeed, experience becomes the point of departure for a feminist critique, one that has learned from Marx that the transformation of our society can only proceed from knowledge of the whole, which itself is not possible without the standpoint of the oppressed. For only from this perspective does totality reveal itself as a false whole.

In the retelling of experiences of violence, fear, anxiety, contradiction, and everyday life, the aim is never merely to tell one's story. For Haug, it is a methodological approach to a collective process of learning that one's own experiences are not so private after all, that what one takes to be intimately one's own bears the marks of society. The truth of what it means *to be made a woman* and *to make oneself a woman* lies precisely within that experiential world and its reflection, in that felt mediation between subject and object which thought can grasp. Her writings occupy this place: between the immediacy of domination—which is never truly immediate—and its conceptual comprehension.

This volume, therefore, begins with a theme at the very heart of Haug's work: experience. The opening text, "The Other Anxiety," traces the gendered structure of anxiety—one of women's most fundamental emotions, at once constraining and self-preservatory. Its central claim is simple yet devastating: while men may fear many things, women above all fear men. Far from irrational, this fear is both justified and confirmed statistically. Men commit nearly all recorded acts of serious violent offenses and homicide, as well as the overwhelming majority of sexual assaults against both adults and children. For women, cohabitation with a man remains one of the most persistent and lethal risk factors—a reality that transforms the private into a site of domination. What is felt as *personal* anxiety is determined by the structure of society. Those puzzled by why women of all ages will declare (half in jest) on social media that they would rather encounter a bear in the woods than a man will find answers in Haug's essay.[1] This gendered anxiety contains both irrational and rational elements. On the one hand, it serves a rational, self-preservatory function that attests to the grim truth of real threat. On the other hand, it disperses indiscriminately across men and nature, while sparing the men whom women invite into their homes and beds. But as the recent Pélicot Trial in France[2] reminded us with cruel perspicuity, there is no *safe space* for women—not even, or especially, within the supposed sanctity of home. Male violence, and the fear it engenders, functions as one of patriarchy's most effective instruments: both subtle and brutal, it compels submission, driving women from public space into the private sphere—often the more perilous realm.

To render such experiences accessible, Haug developed a remarkable new feminist methodology, which she discusses in "Methodological Questions in Everyday Feminist Research." This essay asks what constitutes a specifically feminist empirical method. To this end, Haug discusses possible conceptual frameworks in relation to women's oppression and demonstrates their implications for theory and empirical research. Focusing on everyday life as a problem in Marxism and ethnomethodology, particularly in the works of Antonio Gramsci and Henri Lefebvre, she elaborates three key feminist methodologies: Dorothy Smith's, Carol Gilligan's, and her own method "memory work." While Smith reveals that scientific concepts function as instruments of power that exclude and regulate women—distortions which feminist research must expose—Gilligan, in turn, demonstrates how women are socially prompted to suppress and deny their own knowledge, arguing that liberation requires the collective reappropriation of this voice. After highlighting not only the productive dimensions of these two approaches but also some of their limits, Haug finally turns to her own method.

Memory work is a collective research method that treats experience as the foundation of knowledge. Participants—typically women in Haug's practice, though the method itself is not confined to this group—share memories around a common theme (e.g., anxiety). These memories are written down, shared within the group, and analyzed collectively to trace how experience is constructed. By focusing on the written memory, the method orients inquiry toward the construction of the self: how the memory takes the form it does, what it conceals and what it reveals, and how social structures determine both memory's content and form and self-perception. Broadly, memory work investigates how personality is molded by the very structures that individuals inhabit and help to reproduce. It examines how women live the conditions of existing society that shape both their individuality and their experience.

Memory work arose as a response to traditional research methods, which impose theory onto experience, flattening it through the process of subsumption. Instead, memory work begins with participants' own memories of experiences, thus transforming the researcher herself into the object of research. The process is neither easy nor free of tension. Collective engagement often surfaces conflict, repressed guilt, and the realization that people cling to their existing identities and experiences as if to salvation. Memory work has changed and evolved through its encounters with these difficulties. Its main question is: What forms do individual life processes take? It rests on the premise that each experience constitutes an appropriation of existing social structures, which are shaped by class, gender, sexuality, race, and other factors. Each memory is thus at once singular and a trace of the social whole.

The mediation of the subjective and the objective—how lived experience is unconsciously informed by concepts and presuppositions, and how these formative processes can be theorized and grasped—is also the central concern of the text that follows, "The Relation Between Experience and Theory in Feminist Research." There, Haug begins by inquiring into the nature of experience. At first glance, experience may appear as something authentic and immediate; a safeguard against external influences and deceptions; something that is truly one's own. Yet, Haug insists that the opposite is the case. It is precisely where something is rendered "merely personal" that we should be most suspicious, for it is there that the traces of society are most insistent. Social structures, norms, and relations of domination are reproduced and inscribed within lived experience. Thus, experience cannot be taken at face value in research but must always be critically examined to unfold the ways in which it is socially mediated and ideologically formed.

As the essay argues, women's experiences are frequently diminished, negated by "male abstraction," or dismissed as trivial within both scientific discourse and societal discourse. Such devaluation and exclusion reveal the persistent structural bifurcation between science and the domestic-private sphere—two domains that have been constructed and rigidly hierarchized as opposites.

However, to trace the constitution of gender identity and the social formation of femininity, these seemingly separate spheres—the personal and the scientific, the private and the public—must be brought into relation to show how they mutually constitute and inform one another. Only by uncovering the construction of femininity through conceptual articulation and theoretical reflection on the ostensibly apolitical, everyday personal experiences of women can the ideological structure of gender relations be rendered visible.

What is laid bare in this process is the profound entanglement of domination and subjectivity, an interrelation engendered and sustained by the social division of labour, duties, and responsibilities. Experience thus becomes a site in which relations of power and domination are both inscribed and reproduced, while simultaneously retaining the potential for transformation through critique.

In her writings, Haug has long wrestled with the challenge of capturing experience in thought—of allowing it to speak in its voice without letting its particularity conceal the social structures that shape it from within. This work with experience is not confined to women's immediate accounts but extends to other sources, notably literature. The third text in this volume is devoted to this topic in particular.

The starting point of "Feminist Literature and Working with Female Experience" is the claim that the formation and articulation of female experience is often more easily conveyed through literature than through theory. This is not an evasion of theory, but a treatment of literature as material for social scientific knowledge. Through an analysis of Marge Piercy's *Fly Away Home* and *Braided Lives*, Haug draws lessons about women's subjugation, bodies, abortion, and the family, revealing that while one cannot exist as a conscious, sensuous being without a body, the society in which we live transforms women's body into a prison, which negates the possibility of a conscious and truly human sensuous existence.

Haug's careful reading of these two novels unfolds the struggles and impossibilities of women's individuality. The truth that gaining individuality as a woman requires the abolition of bourgeois family does not immediately translate to experience. In the failed attempt to reconcile desires with societal demands, women reveal the limits of abstract commands of liberation. Haug shows this by turning to the construction of women as social and private subjects with a determinate function in the social division of labour. She traces the collision of desires, wishes, and demands within the ongoing reproduction of oppression. What emerges is not evidence of false feelings, but the insight that the integration of life's hopes for happiness into the form of the private family renders them dull, anticipatory forms of unhappiness—the longing for life transforms into the renunciation of life. This dynamic does not only pertain to women for it is a prerequisite for exploitation and injustice in general. Yet, Haug's analysis also gestures toward the possibility of life without surrender and a body whose sensuality can be lived without being sacrificed, against its will, to further that of another. What is revealed, in short, is the possibility of a life whose very conditions no longer demand women's surrender but allow for self-determination. Given the recent attacks on women's right to bodily self-determination worldwide, and the particularly alarming success of efforts in the United States to roll back the hard-won progress, these reflections are as urgent and relevant as ever.

"Women Live Resistantly" further examines the contradictions inscribed in women's experiences due to the demand to be both fully human (and, thus, actually individual) and simultaneously to dissolve themselves by surrendering entirely to the family.

In dialogue with Marge Piercy, Doris Lessing, Virginia Woolf, Carol Gilligan, Alexandra Kollontai, and Bertolt Brecht, as well as her own life story, Haug explores the blockages that prevent women from resisting the structures that render their individuality impossible. The life of the housewife emerges neither as pure coercion nor free choice, but as the product of contradictory desires that capitulate, unfulfilled. Women's attempts to fulfill their desire for happiness and love lead to a trap, binding them to domestic drudgery and the stultifying routines of private life. In these conditions, women attempt to render family life a counter-world to the rigid and cold structures of capitalist society. These forms of resistance, which Haug describes as turning women into "moral crusaders" against a repressive and damaging form of society, remain ultimately impotent, merely stabilizing the order they seek to challenge. In light of the aforementioned political rollbacks and the attempts to re-idealize traditional gender roles—exemplified, for instance, by the "tradwife" movement—these reflections stand as a warning against regressing from the collective learning processes already achieved by women.

For women, Haug argues, integration into society exacts the price of the self; one cannot integrate without giving oneself up. Their childhood desires are swiftly renounced under the weight of the demands of adulthood, and their pursuits of happiness through love reveal themselves to be traps that stunt their development. The traps hidden in the image of love are shamelessly depicted in popular romance novels, where male violence is reinterpreted as courtship; indeed, even rape is sometimes normalized as a prelude to love and marriage.

The continuity with dark romance plots and recurring romcom formulas is hardly deniable here.

Clinging to love as a possible source of fulfillment is, for Haug, both a sign of domination and a protest against it. Love carries a dual burden: it promises happiness while harboring the danger of self-extinction. Do we seek love only to find unhappiness along the way, Haug asks? The revolt against being a good daughter, a loving mother, and an obedient wife, with all the loving and hating submission it entails, she argues, must be transformed into a resistance that does not merely refuse subjugation but reconstructs love itself such that the prison is shattered.

The demand to rethink love itself may lead one to scrutinize its manifold social and sexual forms. The "political lesbianism" of the 1970s famously understood lesbianism as a political stance involving a conscious break from men. It was not primarily about sexual orientation but about the deliberate choice to prioritize solidarity and emotional bonds among women rather than entering into dependent heterosexual relationships. Haug's article "Lesbian or Heterosexual–Heroines for Our Liberation" alludes to this debate. It revolves around the question of whether differences can be discerned between lesbian and heterosexual heroines in feminist crime novels, which Haug co-edits for the feminist political crime series, *Ariadne*. The essay initially demonstrates the contrasting ways in which these stories represent the lived realities of heterosexual and lesbian women. The worlds of heterosexual heroines appear more deeply shaped by the burdens of everyday life: their relationships with men, children, marriage, and endless responsibilities—circumstances to which they must, in effect, resign themselves. While these novels offer familiar and relatable narratives, Haug states that, perhaps surprisingly, readers nevertheless gravitate more strongly toward the lesbian protagonists, whose lives appear less fettered by such constraints, seemingly allowing a freer relationship to sexuality and desire. Novels featuring lesbian heroines play with alternative forms of female self-determination, solidarity, and pleasure—one that envisions not only individual liberation but also a new political and emotional reconfiguration of love. This reimagining of love—as a site of both personal transformation and social critique—extends beyond literature into the broader terrain of experience. Feminist literature thereby assumes the character of a critical practice that experiments with different forms of living and can transform narrated experience into a means of emancipation.

How emancipation might be achieved, what impedes it, and how the relationship between the individual and society can be understood—these are the questions that fundamentally drive Haug's work and which are directly addressed in "Victims or Agents." The essay is one of her most important and contentious interventions in feminist and Marxist scholarship. In collaboration with Haug, this volume presents a new translation of the essay with the aim of introducing its challenging insights for contemporary feminism to a broader audience.

The argument developed here is that emancipatory praxis demands recognizing that the oppressed—in this case, women—are themselves complicit in the active reproduction of the very structures that subjugate them. To bring this complicity to light is not to assign blame or cast moral judgment, but to illuminate the insidious reach of ideology, which permeates even the most intimate layers of subjectivity. The aim of "Victims or Agents" is to bring to light the process by which domination, itself a product of human actions, shapes subjectivity.

Throughout her writings, Haug relentlessly urges women to take up their own cause: act or be acted upon. This is not a facile exhortation to simply "do something," but a demand to confront the ways in which women participate in the creation and reproduction of the very conditions of their subjugation in capitalist society. From this perspective, emancipation is not reducible to the mere overthrowing of institutions. In keeping with Marx's claim that the dissolution of the proletariat is the dissolution of capitalism, women's emancipation involves their own dissolution. Central to this claim is the Marxist view that social relations, and thus capitalist domination, are a product of our own activity. For Haug, likewise, domination functions through the participation of the oppressed. Women thus occupy a paradoxical position: neither passive victims nor ready-made agents of change, but agents of existing society, nonetheless.

That women are oppressed is indisputable; evidence of their victimhood is ubiquitous. But how can women resist the very oppression whose traces they carry within themselves? The essay outlines two interlocking obstacles. First, the oppressed bear the marks of their oppression. Second, women confront not only external, structural barriers to emancipation but also internal ones that hinder the revolutionary impulse—attachments to private life and relationships, marriage, motherhood, and their historical link to nature. Why, Haug asks, do women participate in these structures that constrain them and whose marks they bear? This participation, she suggests, is rooted in an unconscious secret desire for these oppressive structures—which are appealing insofar as they appear as escape from other forms of capitalist domination, such as wage labour—and constitutes a tacit consent to one's own submission. Oppression that is not enforced solely through external coercion, Haug argues, relies on the consent of those involved.

To the contemporary reader, Haug's argument may sound like victim blaming. After all, who willingly seeks out their own subjugation? Yet, Haug's point is that if women are assumed to be merely victims, how could they possibly transform their condition or participate in its transformation? If women, like all people, are subject to structures that endure only through our constant reproduction thereof, then domination can only be overcome by those who reproduce it. The idea that women can change their conditions presupposes their role in creating the conditions they seek to transform.

If oppression is lived, internalized, and woven into daily existence and the structures of personality, then liberation cannot be imposed from without. In short, women must contend with their complicity in their own subordination. The argumentative framework thus relies on an analysis of capitalist relations, which are often obfuscated in contemporary feminism. That it places women within structures of domination as its victims, but also creators and possible agents of destruction, means that agency is not pre-given. By treating individuals as social categories determined by the form of society, the essay captures both the rigidity of social relations and their possible abolition.

This analysis highlights that feminist emancipation requires the study of our conditions and relations in capitalism in relation to our experiences, but never in such a way that the former is blinded by the latter. It shows that our very actions, positions, and experiences can be obstacles to change. It thus also implies that while feminist theory must draw from experience, it cannot merely rely on *immediate* experience, which can only show one side of this structure: victimhood. Clinging to this side does not promise justice or security, but merely condemns women to existing conditions. The hidden side—that of our agency—is the one that harbors the revolutionary impulse. Only by highlighting this dimension can we stand against our existing selves and with the decline of what is.

"Practice of Critique" addresses the question of self-transformation from yet another perspective. Haug begins by recounting the moments of frustration she experienced working with students admitted into higher education through a second-chance program—individuals shaped by their concrete experience of labour under capitalist conditions—as she sought to make science accessible to them as a tool for understanding their own lives. She describes the difficulties of presenting critique as a weapon for thought: instead of adopting it readily, the students repeatedly resisted, forcing her to reexamine her own assumptions.

Drawing on Karl Marx, Antonio Gramsci, Klaus Holzkamp, and, especially, Bertolt Brecht, Haug elaborates how the process of becoming a researcher of oneself transforms the very meaning of critique. Critique, she argues, is not simply the negation of what exists but a dialectical working-through of the social contradictions sedimented within subjects. In this sense, it is both a dialogical process and an active form of self-engagement—what, following the model of Socratic midwifery, can be conceived as a practice of birthing thought through struggle.

In this sense, critique becomes more than a theoretical exercise: it becomes a transformative activity that joins self-reflection with collective emancipation. To practice critique, then, is to intervene in one's own construction and thereby assume agency over one's own becoming—an often painful but necessary act for liberation.

As already evident, Haug's engagement with Marx and the analysis of labour are crucial to understanding the connection between subjective experience and objective social conditions. In line with the materialist feminist tradition, Haug's reading of Marx exposes an epistemic blind spot: women's labour, though essential to capitalism's functioning, remains largely untheorized.

Even so, Haug's "Feminist Work with Marx" demonstrates the productivity and indispensability of Marx's critique of political economy for feminist theory. Haug reconstructs feminist critiques of Marxism not only to show the continued relevance of Marx's "Theses on Feuerbach" for feminism (as she had also done in her writings on experience) but also to recover from Marx a concept of labour that can ground a theory of a different form of human activity. This, in turn, makes it possible to grasp women's labour in society from a new perspective: not merely as derivative of wage labour, but as a qualitatively distinct form of socially necessary activity that reveals the contradictions of capitalist life.

Haug agrees with feminist critics such as Claudia V. Werlhof and Mariarosa Dalla Costa in noting that women's work remains undertheorized in Marx's writings. Yet, she rejects the claim that this gap is inherent to Marx's concept of labour. Rather, the essay contends that Marx's analyses of capitalist contradictions and the transformation of labour into an alienated activity indicate an emancipatory potential that women, too, can appropriate for their own liberation. Thus, Haug does not discard Marx but works with him, excavating the Marxist categories through which women's subjection and the possibility of transformation can be thought together.

Haug's interpretation highlights that, for Marx, labour is always a contradictory process: both the source of human self-realization and the medium of domination. In the capitalist mode of production, living labour becomes subordinated to dead labour, converting human creativity into a force of alienation. Yet, in this very contradiction resides a possibility: by grasping labour as a historically specific form of human activity—and not as its eternal essence—Marx's work makes it possible to imagine forms of praxis beyond alienation.

Haug thus insists that feminist theory must radicalize rather than reject Marx's critique of political economy. By analyzing how women's unpaid reproductive labour underpins the accumulation of capital, feminism can expose the logic by which capitalism exploits and conceals life-producing activity. The task is not merely to *add* women to Marx's theory but also to transform the very meaning of labour and critique. In doing so, Haug recovers what Marx called "free life activity"—a vision of self-determined, sensuous, and social production—as the ground on which both feminist and socialist emancipation must be built.

A similarly redemptive and critical reading is undertaken by Haug in "Engels' Problem with the Woman Question." On the centenary of Engels' death, she examines whether his *The Origin of the Family, Private Property and the State* still contains untapped conceptual tools for a theory of women's liberation or whether it has instead obstructed such a perspective within the workers' movement. She argues that by conceptualizing historical periods in terms of a shift in the form of domination—from societies regulated by "ties of kinship" to those regulated by labour, property, and class—Engels displaces the analysis of labour in the first phase and of gender relations in the second, thereby rendering women's oppression a systematic blind spot.

Although Engels begins by theorizing production and reproduction of immediate life, he goes on to separate "labour" from "family" in his analysis of capitalist production. As a result, care, nursing, and domestic work fall out of the concept of social labour reduced to the mere organization of biological processes rather than as an integral component of the overall social production. By appraising Engels' account of the transition from hunting to cattle breeding, the essay shows how his formulations efface the complexities of food preparation, care, and livestock management—those activities historically assigned to women.

Yet, for Haug, Engels' reflections hint at a critical insight. In particular, she highlights a far-sighted yet theoretically unpursued passage where Engels deals with the division of household management: only with the rise of monogamous nuclear family does domestic labour become a "private service," excluding women from social production. Engels, however, does not develop this insight into a sustained theory of domestic labour. Working both with and against Engels, Haug insists that this omission has consequences for liberation strategy—consequences that can only be grasped by a theoretical framework capable of analyzing the simultaneous development of the proletariat and patriarchy.

In "The Neoliberal Project," Haug takes up Engels' observation that the capitalist drive toward profit, and thus labour-saving methods and growth, renders time-intensive care and maintenance work a permanent social problem. She develops this line of inquiry through an analysis of the *Courage to Depart* (also known as the Swiss White Paper) authored by leading Swiss economists. She diagnoses a fundamental misconception in the public discourse on work: despite decades of feminist critique, the social concept of labour remains narrowly confined to paid wage labour. Domestic labour, care work, childrearing, and other forms of reproductive labour may be formally acknowledged as "work," yet continue to play no structural role in economic or political theory. This dominant conception of labour, the essay argues, is a male one: it rests on the systematic exclusion of care, nurturing, and reproductive activities and on the delegation of these unpaid tasks to women.

Haug's critique of neoliberal ideology shows how economic domination is cloaked in a rhetoric of moral self-responsibility, suggesting that structural problems can be solved through individual behavior. At the same time, Haug reveals how the dismantling of the welfare state and the deepening of social inequality rely on the availability of women's free labour. That is, women are expected to fill the gaps left by the retreat of public welfare, absorbing the social costs of neoliberal restructuring. Neoliberalism, it follows, is not merely an economic program but a comprehensive social project—one that, with devastating social and ecological consequences, replaces the activity of human beings, as a collective species-being, with the autonomous movement of capital. Genuine social renewal, she argues, can succeed only if gender relations are understood and transformed as a foundational element of economic and political structures. This requires negotiating a new gender contract, one that brings the reproduction of life—education, care, and ecological responsibility—out of the private sphere and into the center of political and social planning.

Haug's call for far-reaching political transformation further unfolds in "From the Fisherman and His Wife" through her reflections on the concept of the *domination knot*. The knot is the intricate interlacing of different threads of domination—visible and invisible—that sustain one another and maintain the fabric of capitalist society. These threads—encompassing wage labour and unpaid labour and their relation to accumulation and profit, the neglect of human development, the invisible work of sustaining human life and nature, and the denial of political participation—are secured through our actions, habits, hopes, dreams, wishes, morals, and common sense.

The domination knot is not merely the interaction of distinct forms of oppression. In this sense, Haug's concept offers both a critical alternative and possible complement to what is now theorized as "intersectionality." Both frameworks share the fundamental insight that relations of domination are not discrete but interwoven, producing complex configurations of power and subordination. Yet, their epistemological and political orientations differ. Whereas intersectionality, as popularized by Kimberlé Crenshaw, employs the metaphor of a traffic intersection to illustrate how multiple axes of oppression—such as race, class, and gender—converge in lived experience, Haug's image of the shoelace knot shifts the analytical perspective from the level of individual positions to that of structural interdependence. Her metaphor emphasizes the tightly bound, mutually reinforcing entanglement of domination, where the strands—capital's profit-driven logic, the invisible labour of social reproduction, the neglect of human development, and political subalternity—do not merely cross but bind.

The difference between these two frameworks extends also to their aims. Much of contemporary intersectional theory focuses on making visible and contesting overlapping forms of discrimination and exclusion within existing social and legal frameworks; its horizon is recognition, representation, and justice within a plurality constitutive of liberal capitalism. Haug's domination knot, by contrast, articulates a transformative materialist critique: it seeks to grasp and ultimately dissolve the systemic interlocking of capitalist, patriarchal, and political domination. Domination, she insists, is tightly intertwined and resistant to unraveling. Multiple threads make it nearly impossible to untangle, and attempts to intervene can backfire. The danger lies in pulling the wrong end, which merely tightens instead of unraveling the knot. Thus, if one tugs at the thread of unpaid labour and demands it becomes paid, the result is not emancipation but the conversion of unpaid labour into waged dependency. The knot, Haug warns, must be undone otherwise. But how? This untying is fraught with complications. For just as laced shoes make walking easier, the domination knot, however constraining, affords stability, comfort, security, even reward. As Haug argues in "Victims or Agents," all forms of oppression presuppose agency of the subjected. Insofar as domination entwines subjugation with rewards and security, loosening the knot threatens to leave one unsupported, like walking with undone shoelaces—freer, yet stumbling. The solution, Haug insists, cannot lie in the selective tugging of individuals' threads. To pull one alone merely tightens the whole; emancipation demands that all be drawn upon at once, that the total knot be unsettled. Only in this simultaneity does the knot begin to loosen, and domination becomes unstable. Recognizing the danger such insecurity provokes, she recalls Brecht's remark that when the ruling class loses its grip, the ruled collapse first. For the untying of the knot not to harden into a new form of paralysis, all must take part in recreating social conditions and remaking everyday life. The goal, therefore, is not the inclusion of marginalized positions within existing structures, but the radical transformation of society itself—an emancipatory project aimed at liberating human capacities from the interlaced constraints of capital, gender hierarchy, and political passivity.

At the end of the essay, Haug returns to *The Fisherman and His Wife* fairytale to demonstrate the doomed fate of one-sided attempts at wish-fulfillment—a mirror image of the effort to break free from domination by pulling on a single thread. The wife, sitting idle in a hovel, forgets her own agency and displaces the fulfillment of her wishes onto her husband. Her ensuing punishment seems to affirm the moral that she ought to remain content in her poverty. The fisherman, for his part, fares little better: the wish is displaced yet again, now onto the division of labour. The social totality becomes harder to discern. Untying the domination knot requires grasping and revealing the intertwinement of different forms of labour that appear divided, as a first step toward emancipation.

In her reflections on the domination knot, Haug gestures toward her conception of a utopia by women for all which she terms the "Four-in-One-Perspective." This vision is elaborated in her book *Die Vier-in-einem-Perspektive: Politik von Frauen für eine neue Linke* [The Four-in-One-Perspective: Women's Politics for a New Left]. For the reader's benefit, we have chosen to include an excerpt from this book under the same title.

Following Marx's insight that the development of each individual is a precondition for the development of all, Haug's utopian vision insists that liberation must entail the unfolding of capacities dormant in each one of us. Emancipation, she insists, cannot be bestowed; it must be enacted by all of us; otherwise, it will be of no consequence to us.

The "Four-in-One-Perspective" envisions a society with a wholly new organization of labour, and thus a new life itself—a new time regime in which human activity is oriented around four interwoven spheres: labour, reproduction, self-development, and politics. Each sphere is allotted four hours, not as a mechanical division of hours, but as a compass for orientation. Labour, the first sphere, names the social work necessary to sustain collective life and secure means of subsistence. The second, reproductive labour, encompasses reproductive work, care, and maintenance, equally essential for society as a whole; this sphere will also be generalized, hence shedding its gendered character. The third, self-development, entails activities for development and enjoyment. And finally, the fourth, politics, which for Haug means collective decision-making. Each member of society must participate in all four spheres. As such, specialization, which today mutilates individuals, is abolished for the sake of the all-round development of each individual.

Haug presents this concrete utopia as a new time regime, where all four dimensions of life are woven together into an alternative model of society. This vision exposes the one-sided development of individuals in capitalism, where life is consumed by labour. Thus, Haug warns that every sphere pursued in isolation becomes reactionary. To the contrary, the Four-in-One-Perspective seeks to alter our society's regime of time. Though not an immediately realizable goal, it serves as a compass for our demands and a basis for critique. It points toward a society in which development does not entail the mutilation of individuals, the one-sided development of some at the expense of others, but a life where the development of each is a condition for the development of all.

The volume concludes with an "Interview with Frigga Haug"—the conversation that gave rise to this project. When we traveled to La Palma to conduct this interview, we did not intend to edit a collected volume of her essays. Yet, the richness of Haug's reflections and experiences—and the striking absence of English translations of her work—made such undertaking seem not only desirable but also eminently necessary. The interview offers both an intellectual and personal retrospective, with Haug reflecting on her life's work, the multiple forms of resistance she encountered in research and daily life alike, and the historical and political contexts that shaped her thinking.

Her reflections delineate a remarkable intellectual and political trajectory: from the controversy surrounding "Victims or Agents"—where she insisted on recognizing women's complicity in domination as a precondition for their possible liberation—to the development of participatory research and memory work and finally to the utopian horizon of the four-in-one-perspective. Throughout, Haug conceives theory not as an abstract exercise but as a *praxis* of transformation: knowledge as collective self-education, politics as shared responsibility, and feminism as a materialist project aimed at reorganizing the social foundations of life.

For some, perhaps, making anti-capitalist politics central to feminism may sound daunting, if not passé. However, contemporary feminism has much to learn from Haug's analysis, which demonstrates that the emancipatory desire to overcome capitalism should become the main objective of feminist thought. This desire requires that we see society with clarity, without illusions, acknowledging the reified conditions under which we live, have become, and must break. Change is brought about by consummating society's contradictions, which are embedded in our own personality structures. Emancipation may thus appear as a progress that we do not intuitively embrace—for it requires acknowledging our hand in domination and aligning with interests which do not serve emancipatory rather than immediate interests. In this way, Haug's departure from the tired claim of women's double oppression—as women and as workers—to refocus our attentions on their double character—as victims and as agents—remains as relevant as ever.

What emerges from the interview is more than a portrait of a pioneering thinker. It constitutes a living archive of Marxist-feminist struggle and renewal. Haug's perspective in our conversation is animated by the conviction that emancipation begins when people become researchers of their own conditions—a principle that weaves together the many threads of her thought.

By Alexandra Colligs and Jeta Mulaj

Notes

1 For a discussion of this debate on Social Media, see, for instance, Marjorie Philibert, "Alone in a Forest: Most Women Would Rather Run into a Bear Than a Man," *Le Monde*, June 21, 2024, https://www.lemonde.fr/en/our-times/article/2024/06/21/alone-in-a-forest-most-women-would-rather-run-into-a-bear-than-a-man_6675309_39.html

2 From 2011 to 2020, Dominique Pelicot from Mazan, France, drugged and raped his wife, Gisèle Pelicot, and invited male strangers to rape her while she was unconscious. Dominique and 50 other men accused of rape were brought to court and convicted in 2024. For more information on this case, see for instance; Ségolène Le Stradic and Catherine Porter, "Pelicot Trial Timeline," *The New York Times*, October 6, 2025, https://www.nytimes.com/2025/10/06/world/europe/pelicot-trial-timeline.html

Translator's Note and Reflection

Cindy Zeiher

Between 2023 and 2025, I was busy translating Frigga Haug's texts for this collection. Having previously translated her work, I thought I knew what to expect. However, it was not long into the translation process that I realized how deftly Haug weaves together so many intellectual threads to make her singular points.

Frigga Haug was already an established activist-academic in Germany when I was still a child, growing up in a working-class, immigrant family under a self-serving, right-wing state government. My own complex and alienating background triggered my interest in trade unionism and feminism. Although committed to unionism, community, and political work, I was struggling creatively at the time and had put that part of my life on hold until later. Haug's *The Four-in-One Perspective: A Utopia by Women, A Utopia for All* text led me to reflect on why this was and why women in particular should relinquish part of themselves to accommodate a chaotic, patriarchal world. Many years later, following motherhood and a change in career and country, I find myself reflecting on Haug's insightful writings and, in particular, how, as their lives unfold, my two daughters now have the privilege of taking for granted some of the wins and attributes of feminism fought so hard for by women such as Haug. Although this transition is welcomed progress, beneath it all lies a certain melancholy regarding the historical ups and downs of feminism and feminists: what is lost or won, and what needs to be preserved or let go. Of course, some things have changed for the better; women can now speak openly on specific topics without being overly burdened by once-held fears. However, self-replicating societal structures through which we express our ideas are still enabling opaque and oppressive patriarchal conditions. Even as I was editing Haug's texts, the world was embracing right-winged politics with a glossy individualist sheen; the USA re-elected a President accused of sexism and misogyny and found liable for rape, while women's labour worldwide continues to be undervalued and taken advantage of. In my "home" country, Aotearoa/New Zealand, a conservative government ruled by three men has repealed existing pay equity for women legislation and replaced a progressive sex/gender guide for state schools with a regressively redacted document of its own. Misogyny post #MeToo remains confident, sexism is still rife, even if more nuanced and individualized; women remain anxious and feel unable to speak out about their experiences for fear of being disbelieved or even ostracized. As military, class, and gender wars are being waged all over the world, we need more than ever an injection of Haug's radical, uncompromising feminism.

Frigga Haug is a force to be reckoned with, strong, and attentive to the conditions in which women in Germany live and seek a way to thrive. She makes it her business to listen to these women's experiences in all their inevitable contradictions and to the anguish they face when trying to articulate these. Moreover, Haug, as a militant pacifist (a position I share), resolutely confronts the consequences of this position be it via personal risk or active opposition. Translating Haug's words, I was struck by her sense of women's precariousness, stress, and anxiety in today's world. As a mother protesting in Berlin during the 1980s, Haug and the collective she was a part of were very much a minority. They brought their children to protests, notwithstanding that such a spectacle went against the grain of "good" mothering. She recalls that when protesting in Berlin against the USA military involvement in Vietnam, she found herself and her children in need of protection from the very power she was critical of, as German Vietnam war supporters began to harass the collective she was a part of. In this way, preserving images of contradiction, Haug offers a powerful insight and questions into the complexities of power and protection.

At the same time, it became apparent during the translation process that Haug was not simply one more pragmatic German Marxist striving for the synthesis of nations. For her, great insights were to be found in myths, legends, and fantasies emanating from everyday life. I read some of these stories to my then-young daughters in order to pass on a part of my German heritage and imagination. Fairy tales and myths are ambiguous, allowing us not only to tap into nostalgia and be transported to alternative worlds but also to reveal both what we lack and what we have become. They mirror our ethics and serve as a testing ground for our sense of fate. Haug understands and recognizes the importance of fantasy. How to handle the horrible kernels of truth it offers, namely that women, despite repeated attempts, struggle to designate a place that is wholly theirs. Translating Haug, I was confronted with a stunning relation concerning myth: myths fail via their contradiction, and this is their very function. To pragmatically do away with myth is borderline stupid, because it is myth that reveals what cannot or does not fit. Haug used myth as a referent, a psychic architecture of literalness which brings the ordinary into a strange world, and vice versa. More than once, she refers to philosopher Ernst Bloch, who dared to imagine a better world, despite living through the trauma of antisemitism, WWI, the Great Depression, the rise of fascism, and several civil wars. For Haug, merging philosophy with Marxism represented not only a possibility for critique but also a clarifier, offering a sense of preparedness for the direction society needed to take and how to harness collective destiny. Haug well knows and appreciates the struggle of living with impossibilities; after all, this is what she spent her academic life chasing. I always noticed that between Haug's words lies a caution: everyone daydreams, even the fascist, the misogynist, the exploiter, or the murderer. She took seriously the writings of Freud particularly his emphasis on dreams as a means of satiating libidinal desire, together with the importance of creating myths to offset desire and thereby live a livable life. She thought it was important for women to reflect critically on their ideas and positions, as these become consequential in enabling them to stand tall and stare straight ahead rather than gaze downwards and thus remain perpetually at risk.

I have always felt admiration for women academics who, at the same time, have embraced the subjectivity of being mothers, commitments that are not mutually exclusive. Caring for others can be an enriching personal experience and need not necessarily encroach negatively on one's intellectual life. Haug was thinking along similar lines, of how one's role as a mother should somehow contribute to social conditions, in her understanding of motherhood as embracing desire as a revolutionary force rather than as acceptance (or otherwise) of essentialist commands. Some of the questions regarding women and labour raised by Haug 30 years ago have not been laid to rest. During the translation process, I was mindful to straddle her firm stance on balancing engagement with enigma as intrinsic to womanhood. Indeed, with the advent of feminism, questions surrounding discriminatory remuneration and ideological myopia regarding women's labour have never been more urgent. Haug picked up on these during the second phase of the feminist movement and attended to matters of politics, motherhood, alienation, and exploitation not only in terms of ideological conditions but also as questions women should ask themselves even when this means confronting the hard and uncomfortable truth of how invested women may be in refusing to ride on the coattails of the patriarchy.

For me, one of the exciting parts of translating Haug's texts is the experience of being transported to a different time and place. The translator's task is, in some ways, to collapse time and distance in order for the author's words to speak in the present, and this is what I attempted to do: Haug's work, her activism, and intellect defy the structures that sought to constrain them. Being German myself, I was greeted with memories—not all positive but confronting and indeed enlightening—concerning certain aspects of German culture and knowledge as an insider-outside is both a blessing and a curse, especially for a translator in this way caught between worlds and languages, where the task is to convert another's images and thoughts into words. For the benefit of non-German readers or those unfamiliar with specific historical events and geographical sites, I have included translator's notes in Haug's texts regarding geographical and historical context, either bracketed or as footnotes. Haug's many references to novelists have, when not already translated, been preserved in her own words.

Translating Haug's many texts has proved tremendously rewarding, almost as if they were being written now. It has been a pleasure and an honor to be involved with this collection of texts and to bring a portion of Haug's oeuvre to the English-speaking world. I thank her for trusting me with the task of translation, as well as co-editors Jeta Mulaj and Alex Colligs, for their patience, steadfast collaboration, attention to the details of editing, and overseeing this incredible collection of essays which can now be shared with the non-German speaking world as well as a new generation of feminist activist-thinkers. It has been such a pleasure to work with you all.

Cindy Zeiher
Ōtautahi/Christchurch, Aotearoa/New Zealand
August 2025

Chapter 1

The Other Anxiety

On the Genderedness of Emotion[1]

Frigga Haug

I once participated in a television program on female anxiety. It commenced with the camera being directed toward a very dark park, with a more precise gaze focused on the narrow bend of a small path, initially unnoticed in the darkness of the park. A woman then entered the scene. Her sudden appearance struck the spectator like a forbidden sign: This is the wrong place for a woman to be at night, alone. The camera immediately enhanced the realization of this "wrongness." It showed her panicking face, large fearful eyes, attentively listening to something. In the background, the sound of her high-heeled shoes clicking on the cobblestones. She hastened her pace. Still, she seemed overly attentive to noise, which sounded like a heart beating. She hastens her pace even more, her eyes in terror, sweat forming on her brow. Under the unmistakable sound of her heartbeat emerges a simultaneous step, stronger and quite different from her clicking shoes. A man's step. The camera leads your gaze behind the woman, who has started to run, suddenly coming to a halt at a man's shoes, feet, and legs. The camera chases his pace, fastening back to the woman. She is running now. However, the distance between them becomes shorter. She will never make it. Now he has reached her, rips her shoulder, and turns her around. He opens his other hand, and innocently, there lies a car key, which he hands her. Here, you feel immense relief because the scene was a harmless gesture of care; you feel shame because you and the woman have almost become hysterical without reason. Moreover, you feel annoyed and cheated because, you know, there *was* a reason. Something is wrong. The scene was not altogether about care and protection.

Preliminary Remarks

Here, I would like to illustrate how memory work proceeds alongside anxiety. I will start by situating the landscape of anxiety. I will then discuss theories of anxiety and turn to memories of anxiety in the body to develop some general theses based on these findings. I relate these to child development and examine the contradictions girls encounter growing up. In the third section, I move to another country and culture, Canada, and try to show the net woven out of fear, gender, and race. The topic of female anxiety allows me to turn to psychology and cultural studies.

DOI: 10.4324/9781003480143-1

Moreover, a report on a long-term study I conducted on anxiety should provide us with the possibility to learn about memory work as a process toward insights into the comparative and well-known theories in the field of anxiety. I intend for anxiety to be understood as both simultaneously cross-cultural and critical.

The Concept and the Sample

We commence with the problem of translation both scientifically and in everyday language because there is no adequate translation for the German term *Angst*. Even studying the different possibilities of translating the terms fear, anxiety, and *Angst* leaves us somewhat at a loss, mainly because their specific meanings melt into each other.[2]

First, I offer data on the empirical study. The research group began with approximately 50 women attending the women's study program at the University of Hamburg. The women were from various occupations, including homemakers and professionals such as nurses, librarians, teachers, theologians, social workers, and unemployed women with no unique background. Some were retired. Women's interests tended to focus on the general issue of anxiety; thus, the range of our sample was broad, both in age (ranging from 20 to 60 years) and in professional/personal background. The study continued for four years and resulted in vast qualitative material consisting of 83 narratives of experiences of anxiety. Also, 11-year-old boys and girls from a public school wrote 32 essays as we attempted to collect anxiety experiences from a developmental-gendered perspective.

The Landscape of Anxiety

Upon reflection, most of us can appreciate that anxiety is a memory reaching so far back into the present that it almost feels like a natural condition, always preparing to disturb body and soul. Very early in childhood, there is a fear of the dark; then, such a fear might develop into one of heights and depths or speed. As one develops, a fear of the public, of the unfamiliar, of change might manifest. Fear hinders us, attacks us, and keeps us under its spell. Anxiety, which we feel we must flee, forces us to find refuge, a home. In this way, anxiety becomes convenient as it accompanies the path of women into protected areas, which might hinder the steps women need to take for change. Therefore, anxiety is an important issue for women.

From the beginning of our research, we found the field occupied by rather strange and (for us) difficult-to-understand emotions, connotations, and stories. For example, one of Grimm's fairytales (which was so fascinating to Bloch), *The Story of a Boy Who Went Forth to Learn What Fear Was*,[3] deals with a young man who set out to learn about fear. He never experiences fear; he is not afraid of white figures at night, nor spooks, hanged men, large black cats, or dogs with glowing chains; he is not afraid when his bed drives on its own or hurls him out. He even feels nothing when he is confronted with halves of corpses, crossbones, and skulls. On the contrary, his productive mind is stimulated, and he positions skulls to bowl them over. The churchyard or any other gruesome place at night does not garner any feeling of fear; even the cold corpse, whom he takes into bed to warm him, cannot make him afraid. Every production of horror is met with his readiness to help, or, if his life is in danger, he can competently overpower those who should make him afraid. His longed-for horror only eventuates when his wife has a bowl of cold, living, wriggling fish poured over him (she does not do it herself but asks a maid to do it because she is, of course, a princess).

Many sophisticated discussions of this fairytale have been written to date. For the most part, the central idea is that it must be a fairytale about the Age of Enlightenment because fear and superstition belonged to the Middle Ages. Nevertheless, we can say that they are still felt as absence, a sort of alienation from nature that can only be met by confronting life and death. It has been interpreted as a story of the prosperous bourgeoisie, who appropriate and dominate nature, overpower dark riddles and superstition at the price of one's alienation from nature. To be human would then mean to regain one's naturalness, which necessarily includes anxiety and horror. This discussion does not sound strange or old-fashioned to women's ears; our problem is that as soon as one thinks about oneself as a woman, a significant leap is made because the world of pure rationality is unattainable, even if such rationality is a questionable goal. Somehow, we all still live in the Middle Ages of anxiety, confronted with numerous dangers and fears.

Once you start researching anxiety, you find it suddenly everywhere: in politics, in newspapers, in flyers that try to offer us advice, in films, and so on. We read sophisticated essays on a general fear of death and, of course, fear of ecological catastrophe, as well as and especially the fear of all "others," of racism, of a new growing fascism. Strangely enough, there exist long articles dealing with anxiety as a means of educating and controlling people—that is, a certain amount of anxiety is needed to behave appropriately, to pay your taxes, not to drive too fast, to keep a well-functioning family, and so on. Wherever you look, you find the strangest opinions on anxiety, thousands of books, and above all, such opinions seem very confident about what anxiety consists of and where one is likely to contend with it. Upon appearance, anxiety is both too vast and superfluous to warrant any further study.

At this conjuncture, we started to brainstorm about anxieties, which gave us the impression that there is nothing that cannot be the source of anxiety and that even opposite reasons—such as being alone or not being alone; being seen or not being noticed at all, and so on—were understood and even shared by everybody in the group. There was no specific method for collecting data on anxiety. So, simultaneously, we studied theories on anxiety. To enable us to couch our work in theory, I will briefly summarize only two schools of thought that are in opposition: psychoanalysis and behavioral theory.

Theories of Anxiety

Psychoanalysis

The most provocative here is Freud. In his early writings, he considers *Angst* to be the effect of unsatisfactory sexuality. He looks at bodily symptoms of anxiety: vertigo, sweating, trembling and shaking, exaggerated heartbeats, difficulties with breathing, and so on. From here, he derives that there is obviously "blocked" excitement, an excessive energy waiting to be released. Without further delay, Freud thinks that there might be something wrong with sexual life; for him, anxiety emerges from frustrated excitement from unsatisfactory sexual intercourse. Women, in addition to this, may experience virginal anxieties because they might not be able to imagine what sexual life is like and are, therefore, unable to handle their excitements. Both sexes suffer from inaction and, above all, from interrupted intercourse, which was, at that time, the typical method of preventing pregnancies.[4]

It is so easy to laugh and dismiss this since it would mean that sexual intercourse would always be satisfactory for women if there were no interruptions and that anxieties about unwanted pregnancies cease upon the introduction of the contraceptive pill. It is easy not to see the originality and usefulness in Freud's ideas, which should be retrieved, especially two pivotal assumptions: first, that the manifestation of anxiety, even in its most extreme presentation, would not be a disease or hysterical but simply typical and following certain practices; and second, the origin of anxiety does not originate in one specific place or cause but emerges from common forms of social and sexual practices of human beings. Freud, of course, neither assumes gender relations as one of domination nor does he think that all social relations could be fundamental for developing anxieties, which both had to be worked through and included in his schema of anxiety as a materialization of mass social practices.

In his later writing, after the experience of the First World War, Freud abandons the idea that one suffers from too little satisfaction and instead positions anxiety between life and death. Anxiety thus becomes the answer to a threat of danger, which the ego cannot handle. This is an interesting elaboration of the contradiction of anxiety, especially in the context of our research on female anxieties. While I will not go into the details of the different instances of psychic apparatuses here, it is important to note that anxiety arises if contradictory demands present themselves because the ego does not find any way through. In this way, the subject is not suffering displacement or repression as a source of anxiety but rather, inversely, an anxiety manifesting from displacement. This also allows us to think that those anxieties that individuals name as such are placeholders for something else. Refraining from jumping to interpretations and instead focusing on those contradictions that people act out would be more helpful. Here, we start to search for experiences of socially given contradictions from the situatedness of women. We hope to be able to include the possibility that social demands that appear unambiguous might well be contradictory and thus a source of anxiety.

Behavioral Theories

Most irritating in behavioral theories is the total lack of interest in the possible reason(s) for anxiety. Anxieties are presumed to function as a disorder, a state that we should get rid of, or which function as a social necessity to maintain decorum. The therapist's main principle is that humans should be able to function. Behavioral science is, above all, about learning, so the question is, which human practices best deal with danger and conflict and can be a substitution for better practices? This idea becomes more convincing as you remember that we all spontaneously develop ways of dealing with anxious situations precisely as behavioral therapy recommends. For example, you might promise yourself something special if you succeed in walking home on your own at night for two blocks, cautiously approaching a dog bit by bit, speaking in front of a smaller then bigger and larger audience, and so on. In these ways, adaptive behavior therapy recommendations appear to duplicate everyday life practices. The uneasiness we feel might come from different sources, and we might not especially appreciate such practices where we try to outsmart ourselves. Theoretically speaking, behavior theories have no space for the idea that anxieties might answer (or respond) to something beyond the obvious, that anxiety might be justified and protective, and that the central implicit assumption about anxiety has been wrong: that anxiety comes from a false perception and thus that re-education enables us to function healthily in a world full of contradictions, domination, violence, and oppression. The presumption is that we would like to function undisturbed in such a society. So, studying behavioral theories, especially those relating to anxiety, has been helpful because they have taught us how to deal with ourselves in everyday life and, as researchers, help clarify our research goal. We did not want to function and fit within society but rather to develop capabilities to change the conditions to which we react with anxiety. We offer that the main difference was to challenge behavioral theory's perception of society, which is often understood as akin to nature (or natural) to which we should adapt. In our case, a world inhabited by humans could be improved rather than adapted to.

Our Research

We started our research by remembering scenes of anxiety at a very general level, by writing "once, when I was afraid." The starting point of writing down understandable, multidimensional, and astonishing scenes led us to concentrate on three main fields of research:

1 Unanticipated anxieties concerning the production of emotion,
2 Unanticipated anxieties concerning the politics of emotions, and
3 Anxieties of the body within gender relations of emotions.

If you compare these fields of study with other research on anxiety, our positioning of anxiety within understandings of production, sex/gender, and politics is the first result of our study as well as (and at the same time) the beginning of each subsequent step of research.

Fear for the Body in Gender Relations

Before presenting and analyzing the written scenes of anxiety with which we commenced, it is important to discover the commonsense reactions of the group so that, if necessary, they, too, can become the subject of discussion. If this is not done, views that derive from the familiar but whose assumptions have not been examined try to impose themselves, hidden in plain sight. Moreover, suppose there is a lack of consistent critical engagement. In that case, we pass up the opportunity to learn something from ideas commonly held but less commonly scrutinized about cultural hegemony and the power of dominant theories circulating in everyday life. Here, we can be sure that in every woman's group, there will be a (sometimes unspoken) consensus that women are afraid of men, of male violence, of encountering them in the dark, of their loud voices, their dominating demeanor. This feeling is so powerful that it seems almost superfluous to study such anxiety, to be astonished by it, and even to appeal to women to overcome their fears. After all, it is well known that in Germany, a woman is raped every four minutes; in the U.S., the time gap is even shorter. In other words, women's anxiety is tangible; dealing with it successfully can only result from the re-education of men or training women in self-defense. Women's anxieties are related to the aggression of men compared to women's more significant physical weakness. Accordingly, when we decided to investigate women's anxieties, we were not surprised to discover that many anxieties are inscribed in this space: women are at the mercy of men. However, on the other hand, the problem remained of persuading others that such anxieties were worthy of study.

Because we all recognized that it is realistic to be afraid of men, especially in the dark, further questions and analysis seemed beside the point. Conversely, we had assumed that anxiety could only be theorized if it were a fantasy, something imagined, exaggerated, or unrealistic—if it were an abstract theoretical construct. The fact that the perception and analysis of reality might be the source for further theoretical understanding of domination was initially overlooked. This was something we, as researchers, had to relearn.

At this conjuncture, I offer one such scene written by a young woman:

The Underground Shaft

It had only been a short time since she had moved to the city; she planned to take public transport home that night after a concert. She liked to go out on her own in the evening, but today, she was uncomfortable about setting out alone without a partner—it was already very late and hardly anybody was on the streets. The others who had been at the concert now scattered in all directions; it was likely that nobody else would be taking the same subway as her. She stood alone before the subway tunnel entrance, afraid to walk down. In front of her, she had an overview of what was happening and could look back occasionally. She would not know what was behind the next bend in the subway tunnel. In addition, she might easily find herself stuck there, with no means of escape or return. She was furious because she felt dependent. She was not making any progress in her journey at all. She did not want to wait any longer to see if other people might arrive with whom she could safely go down to the platform below. So, she plucked up the courage and descended the staircase. It was a horrible feeling to go along the well-lit passage and gradually move closer to the bend. The more she left the entrance behind, the more she felt herself delivered into the unknown. Just one step behind the bend, nobody could see her and help her. She feared the first moment of panic that would come when she caught her first glimpse of the passage behind the bend. The moment of checking was about whether everything was clear or whether a man was lurking with his back to the wall. Moreover, what if there really was a man leaning against the wall? She knew this feeling from when a man was approaching her in the street at night or when a drunken man bumped into her.

For a very short time, her heart misses a beat in shock.

Imagining this moment frightened her. She felt helpless and lonely, like an animal driven into a corner. When other people were nearby or when she was with a girlfriend, she did not allow herself to be harassed. She swore or yelled back. She hated having to lower her eyes out of caution. When other people were around in the subway, she would struggle to retain her power. Whenever a man looked at her, she would stare motionless into his eyes until he had to lower his own. Sometimes, men smiled when they tried to withstand her gaze. She did not smile back. Sometimes, this was not easy. Then, she would think of an abusive word and would quickly remind herself that this was not a game.

Just before she reached the corner of the bend, her anxiety was so great that she turned around and ran back to the entrance as fast as she could. As she ran, her anxiety increased. She now felt she was being followed. She felt that she was involved in an insane, self-induced panic.

Back on the street, she thought for a moment that she would only get home again if she took a taxi. However, she did not want to take a taxi. If she did not get home the ordinary way, she felt she would never be able to manage this again. She would think twice about going out alone again. She was still unfamiliar with the bus system in Hamburg. So, she just walked around searching for a bus stop. When she found one, she checked the timetable and saw that the last bus had gone. She felt desperate. While she stood wondering what to do, she saw women and men walking toward the Tube station. She followed them in the hope of being able to walk along the passage at the same time as them. They were all going the same way. With a feeling of relief, she went down the steps with them. There were many people on the platform. She felt happy and could scarcely believe that a few minutes earlier, she had been in the street alone and in utter despair. At all events, she would carry some CS gas (teargas). On straight roads, it was reassuring to have her finger on the trigger and know that she could spray it at someone. She still felt anxiety when approaching the corner of the Tube.

Her moment of terror nevertheless remained.

To avoid the pitfalls of empathy, that is, simply reexperiencing the experiences of others, we begin to create distance by posing simple questions to the story. This does not mean we avoid meaning and interpretation, but it is important to note what has already been written. The analysis of a text is a process of deconstruction. The aim is not simply to follow the suggested meaning that the writer has conveyed in the text, which we can easily supplement for ourselves, but to clear a path for new and surprising ideas. Instead, we look for those elements that make up a story in a different light, to reassemble the story in different ways, or to make any gaps, ruptures, or contradictions visible. The analysis of the text by reading against the intended meanings in response to specific questions also serves a further purpose: those various constructs the writer creates about herself, other people, or the subject matter can be made visible via intelligent questioning.

In the present case, our first question was: What does the writer describe as anxiety? What does she claim to be afraid of? Even this simple question makes something she had taken for granted—her fear of men—seem less clear-cut. She is afraid to walk around a corner, and she is afraid of this moment of terror. These two anxieties overlap; they are so great that she fails to describe what she might find around the corner. We hear that a man might be lurking, but not what she expects this man to do. She goes to far greater pains to describe the brightly lit passage and the approach of that corner. We all know this scene from countless horror movies, and this playing on people's nerves is a familiar trope among filmmakers. Even if such images do not necessarily trigger feelings of anxiety, they may well intensify them. Since they are familiar with films, fairytales, or television, we concluded that it was important for our research into anxiety to examine how the imagination is produced, illustrated, and reinforced, among others in mass media. In other words, anxiety must be understood *inter alia* as a cultural product.

Our second question ponders what anxiety relates to, how anxiety is socially constructed as well as constructed by the narrator. While the answer to this question yields a picture that is not conscious for the most part, it is still no less effective in governing the author's actions. She describes anxiety in the context of loneliness, or more precisely, of non-sociability. This anxiety is directed at men as soon as she is not a part of a group. She feels safe in every group, whether concertgoers whom she does not know or other young people, whom she also does not know. She explicitly describes men in groups as gender neutral (as men and women); the group is on the lookout to keep danger at bay. As soon as men appear in anonymous crowds—on the bus, for instance—control is extinguished. We learn this from the interpolated scene: that she becomes the target of men's arrogant, violent glances.

If the crowd protects her, she can play with resistance and return their gaze. This act prevents any misdemeanor. It is social, a mode of defense, and not peaceful communication. If a woman and a man meet, the writer tells us, this does not lead to an innocuous social interchange but to violence. Thus, the words "a man or a drunk" are juxtaposed interchangeably, proving that we deal with beings not in control of their senses, especially if their peers do not control them. As a woman, she feels at their mercy. Moreover, she is reduced to mere nature as soon as she lowers her gaze, for she abandons control of her body. Alternatively, she is defenseless and at the mercy of the male gaze. Such nature condemns women to passivity; it prevents her from describing what the lurking man wants from her. Her expectation of what awaits her around the corner is not based on direct experience and is therefore not susceptible to interventions at the level of experience. Instead, it feeds on other experiences where arrogant men gaze at her aggressively. By experiencing every glance from every man as a potential act of violence, she intensifies her fear of the unknown man at whose mercy she finds herself.

However inclined we may be to sympathize with her imaginative construct, we cannot ignore the fact that there is something monstrous about thinking of men's place in the social world exclusively in terms of protection and control and considering the encounter between the sexes as entirely a matter of brute force.

Although already answered in many ways within the last context, this brings us to our third question, which considers how the "other person" is constructed.

Our fourth inquiry relates to the construction of the self. The writer presents herself as a resister and an active and alert woman. Nevertheless, her construction of the scene leaves her with no possible course of action in practice. Even her planned purchase of teargas will prove of no avail since the cause of her panic does not come to meet her on the open street directly but is instead always lurking in anticipation around the corner. Moreover, her fear of fear itself cannot be combated with an object. Her thoughtful strategy of going around the corner accompanied by other people is not one that will conquer her fear but instead serves as an evasion. Indeed, she foresees that if things go on like this, she will soon be unable to go out alone again. In several daily life scenes and contexts, we found this repeated construction of an unnamed evil that somehow emanates from individual men and renders women incapable of action. Here, women experience themselves as sexual beings, as "nature," rather than as human beings encountering other human beings. In these imagined scenes, each man is also reduced to mere "nature" and hence to violence. The scenes are intensified by the elaboration of women's inability to act. In the one described above, the idea that the man is not only lurking behind the corner but also, once she has gone down the stairs, could cut off her retreat. In another narrative, a woman describes lying in bed in her room, imagining what might happen if she went to work in an unfinished office on an isolated building floor. In her mind, she runs through every possible escape route away from an imagined man. She pictures herself just managing to reach a door. However, the corridor is too long, or the door cannot be opened quickly enough, or she cannot negotiate the stairs fast enough, and so on, until she ends up lying in bed, trembling, bathed in her perspiration, her heart racing, unable to go to work at all.

Even with a large amount of empathy for female anxiety regarding male violence, we must admit that most women's fear and anxiety operate without personal experience. For this to occur, the sexes interact in a multifield of social situations; they even live together, so this fear of men must be limited so as not to incapacitate women totally, yet remain capable of being appropriated at any time, thereby threatening the whole social situation of women.

Anxiety in the Dark

Taking a further step forward, we, as researchers, attempted to shed more light on this unspeakable threat by concretizing the question more precisely. Everyone understood from their own experience that the worst anxieties about men arose when in the dark. In such narratives, we hoped to uncover women's anxieties in the earlier scenes more specifically and precisely. Almost any woman could recognize and write these scenes about the dark. Surprisingly, the narratives were all similar, and women shared high degrees of subjective identification. However, even though women knew exactly what it was like to be "in the dark," our analysis still produced some surprising results. For example, in one scene, a woman talks about escaping from a constricting social situation and gaining freedom in nature.[5] Almost at once, she experienced the trees seeming too tall, the wind tremendously blustery, the rain beating down heavily, the fog scarily uncanny, and so on.

Deriving from a confusion between nature without men and the fear of masculine "nature," we were able to arrive at the following theoretical formulations.

For women, there is no social space in which they can be free, and this is why anxiety develops. Such a lack of position leads women to search for freedom in something else, namely, nature—a freedom which they eventually find is too much for them. This new anxiety overwhelms them, and resistance to it drives them toward an individual quest for more suitable living spaces that are ideally outside of society. We had initially assumed that fear of darkness would naturally lead us to statements about fears of masculine violence. Although everyone was quite sure that even scenes about fear of nature were "basically" anxieties about men, it was in the darkness that man was lurking; the trees, wind, and fog were merely signs of man. We soon began to realize that we were not so much concerned here with individual men but with men as the agents of social structures and models for civilization in which women have been assigned unacceptable positions in sexual relations.

Further scenes about fear of the dark contain men or the idea of men lurking in the darkness. At the core of her terror is a woman's anxiety that she is not ready to fight for her life. Instead, we find attempts to achieve sexual neutrality: women conceal their hair beneath a boy's cap, stride with a masculine gait, try to appear manly in a sleeping bag, and think of themselves as plain in the hope of escaping notice by looking unattractive and unfeminine. In all these scenes, the nature of a woman's fate is one where she becomes disembodied. Since such scenes contain no society and no social space worth aspiring to, there is also no possible partner. Women are as lost as they are in nature. Her own "nature" is her existential problem, which restricts her scope for action and where numerous extraordinary incidents disempower her.

One difficulty with working with such scenes about women's anxieties is that it is not imaginary: our societies do contain men who rape and murder women. With such images before their eyes, images that the mass media constantly adds further fuel to, it seems to us that it is normal for women to feel anxiety when they meet men—and more so when men have the opportunity to act free from supervision by others of their kind. This convenient coincidence reveals that the actual process is much more complex. In every social situation, women can feel themselves reduced to their bodies and attempt to use their anxieties to help them escape from the social realm. The problem turns out to be much more deeply anchored in sexual relations in general and in how women are positioned in them.

It frequently happens during memory work that one reaches a point where the analysis of a scene points beyond the horizon of what has been initially thought. Even so, one seems unable to progress in traversing one's fear. This is the case with the fear of men, who constantly slip from one's grasp. In my experience, it is often helpful to move onto a different terrain at such moments.

One option is to look at additional theories on the same topic, hoping that criticism will enable us to make a breakthrough. Another is to interrupt the process of collecting individual testimony and insert a phase in which we explore the socio-economic conditions in which women experience anxiety. A third possibility is to look at fairytales, myths, and images, the material of the imagination. Every path leads somewhere useful. In the present instance, we try one after the other. We ask what role is played in our society by women's bodies and women's "nature," both of which are crucially the starting point, the source, and heart of anxiety. Which contradiction cannot be solved but must be avoided by anxiety?

Women's Bodies in Society

In the journal *Critical Psychology*, a creative Marxist attempt to found a "new" psychology,[6] the decisive distinction between animals and humans has been identified in the fact that the development of the species no longer occurs at the expense of the individuals (as it does if, for example, an animal, like the hare, which is prey for others, begets numerous offspring several times a year; the species survives even if many individual hares die) but depends instead on the development of the individual. This is explained by the ability of human beings to make history and create their world. This arises from objectified labour, language, concepts, and so on; in other words, every individual faces the task of appropriating his/her/their humanity so that humanity can survive humanly.

Inherent in these statements is human reproduction, a process shared by us and the hares, which has been elegantly put aside through neglect. Although all the statements about essential human energies are undoubtedly valid, they bypass the question of how the reproduction of the species is to be regulated in a specifically human manner. At this point, we meet a curious silence, even though it is evident that this aspect of humanization is acted out at the expense of women: physically, morally, and above all, as far as the "appropriation of essential human energies" is concerned. Women know this, but they deny it since they perceive themselves as human beings. They must meet life's various social and historical demands and maintain and protect their bodies for this task to keep them healthy and in readiness. That means that for a certain period, at least, they must also prevent reproduction and live with the countless signals unconsciously and semi-consciously inscribed in society. One such relevant social value is morality in its significance for women. However, even though the prevention of reproduction is one of the aspects of women's behavior that is taken for granted and even though it determines women's emotional world, by the same token, women must be prepared and willing to accept the task of becoming enthusiastic mothers with all the consequences that this entails for their lives and their life-plans. For example, they may always act on the assumption that real life will begin afterwards, that, in effect, they have many lives to live out.

We may perhaps describe this position accurately by saying that women find themselves subject to their bodies. They must act as dutiful overseers of their bodies. At the same time, they realize that these overseers have almost no power—either concerning physical pleasure, their protection, or even their role in the reproduction of humankind. Hence, they incur guilt on every side. Women's fear of men, as also fear about their bodies, must be enormous; what it expresses is that women's entire bodies, their senses, and their whole lives are at the mercy of this reproductive task.

Furthermore, it means that women have no control over their living conditions. They neither "take collective action" to "achieve such control"[7] nor can they do so in the situation prevailing in our societies. We can readily see that the reproduction task is one that they must both desire and fear and that they live within a system complete with contradictory signals. It is not usually thought that to be human is to have too many children in what may well be deprived social circumstances, nor is it held to be feminine to have absolutely no children at all. Society continues to uphold the social rules that assert that sexual behavior outside certain specified conditions is indecent and depraved, and simultaneously that in other specified circumstances, the same behavior is unique and wonderful. (More could be gleaned about these contradictory expectations from a study of the social and individual attitudes to both male and female homosexuality.)

Similarly, the bigoted discussion about the abortion laws should also be reexamined in this context. A light could also be shed on the vulgar (and incorrect) psychoanalytic interpretation that has once again gained currency among men and according to which women's sexual anxieties or fear of rape spring from their intense desire and longing for the very things they resist. The force of this thesis can be understood as an expectation imposed on women, not as a desire they possess.

In the history of humankind, the contradiction about women's bodies sketched here points to immutable constraints and socio-political and cultural deficiencies in the historical relations between the sexes. The problem of human reproduction calls for self-evident values that must be fought for culturally. They require, among other things, the overthrow of our system of morals. Perhaps we do not only lack the experience but also the fantasy to develop intervening utopias. What would we see as a specifically human way of reproduction and an adequate moral and cultural system? In our situation, society's patriarchal development implies a colossal waste of natural resources; women are among those wasted resources in this process. At the stage reached by our civilization, the efforts to develop a human way of reproducing the species seem to have been thought of as individual problems and, hence, have been delegated to individual women. At the same time, on the cultural level, expectations are safeguarded by a network of contradictions that drives the anxieties that reproduce the system. The anxiety that women are forced to develop becomes existential and thus prevents them from recognizing their problems as problems of humanity as a whole. They are thereby prevented from even thinking of alternative approaches.

Anxiety about One's Self

Let us change course once again and return to the anxiety experienced by women in sexual relationships and in a cultural system that semi-consciously fuels this anxiety in a contradictory fashion in the service of its reproduction. We now encounter the problem not only that men can represent a threat to women in reality, but that women themselves grow into society in such a way that they learn to fear men at the same time as they learn to come closer to them and to submit to them. Thus, they acquire the ability to act, simultaneously blocking every escape route.

How is this being achieved? At this point, we each wrote scenes about anxieties concerning oneself. This approach derives from the impression that grew from our work up to now and the conviction that when women express anxieties about their bodies, the entire person is at stake. The following scene might be historical for many readers today, but it still shows emotions and actions that are quite understandable.

A Midnight Cycle Ride

It was immediately after the Currency Reform in 1948, a magic word that seemed like the incarnation of all sorts of promises for her. She was 11 years old, and her sister was 13. In Leipzig, the first fair—another "sparkling" word—was being put on, and her mother wanted to take the opportunity to travel through all the Allied Zones to visit her parents in Berlin since she had not seen them for years, not during the war. There was no way of travelling from the village she was living in—however, a bus left at midnight from one of the neighboring villages. To get there took over half an hour on foot—too far in the dark and with luggage. So, the plan was that their mother would take the luggage on one bicycle, and she and her sister would ride on a second one. On the way back, the two girls could have a bicycle each. Of course, they would ride back quickly—it was already very late, and their two small brothers were left sleeping alone at home. She was very proud that she was indispensable to this plan, which seldom happened since her mother usually worked out her plans just with her sister.

The journey there went quite smoothly. They rode in the pitch-black darkness through puddles and potholes in the road—the carrier she was riding was as challenging as ever, and she longed for the moment when she would at long last be able to ride alone. Together with their mother, they waited for the bus at the chestnut tree in the other village. However, a few drunks were wandering around and pestering them. Their mother became uneasy and sent them off on the return journey before the bus arrived when the men were not looking. They raced off—the thrill of the dark and the importance of their excursion had now shrunk somewhat, thanks to the danger they felt pressing in on them from behind. She kept looking back. As she did so, she caught sight of some bicycle lights and heard voices swearing at them—the voices of the men they had eluded. They were now in full flight; the men raced after them, and despite their drunken state, they caught up with them quickly, making much noise. The girls pushed down on the bike pedals as fast as they could—they ought to put their bike lamps out since they were just illuminated targets. However, the distance between them was already so small that they would never have managed to stop, undo the dynamos, and still make their getaway. They could already hear them panting behind them, and she felt that she was moving weightlessly and could not go on. "Quick, get into the ditch!" her sister cried—and disappeared from her side. She also threw her bicycle into the ditch on the other side and jumped in after it. It was all wet, and she was holding on to the nettles above her for protection when she heard the furious voices of the men above her. They had stopped, having lost sight of their quarry. She pressed against the ground and held her breath, although she wanted to scream from fear and was also afraid for her sister since she somehow imagined that they were after her because she was still too small.

Much later, she heard her sister calling her quietly. Stinging from the nettles, her feet soaked, she clambered, pulling her bicycle behind her. The physical pains filled her with tentative pride for having managed to escape. They decided to ride back into the village to look for their mother or seek out those they knew. Somehow or other, she had expected the men chasing them to reappear. However, another man saw them, loaded them and the bicycles into his delivery van and drove them home.

She felt terrible that she could no longer prove to her mother that she was grown-up and could cycle in the dark, but she also felt there was some justice because she was now allowed to go in a car for her safety.

Methodological Interlude

As illustrated above, we usually approach such scenes with an interrogation that one might find in teaching the study of texts in school. That is to say, we design a set of questions and apply them to the text. A practical method has been to start by compiling lists in columns with straightforward information about, for example, the narrator's actions, actions of others, feelings, and interests. In the second stage, we move on to more complex issues dealing with the construction of the self, the construction of others, or the objects concerned, questions that involve some measure of synthesizing. In the case of the initial question, we enter words that occur in the text, while in the second stage, those words actually used are avoided; similarly, there should be a higher degree of abstraction. The breakdown of the scene into such columns typically brings an immediate insight. For example, one can see how someone can be completely immersed in multiple emotional situations or describe no feelings at all. You can also see the extent to which someone takes action, whether the other participants in the scene behave passively, and so forth. The breakdown of the text into columns is simply a tool, though one that precedes the creation of an analytic, reconstructive text about the scene. It is very illuminating to analyze the language used in the scene, which at this stage has barely been tried with these scenes about anxiety. Our more than a decade-long experience with memory work enables us to conclude tentatively that for most of their experiences, most women only have a borrowed language at their disposal. Moreover, even on the matter of feelings, which are supposed to be the unique terrain of women, there is a vast linguistic deficiency. Clichés are typical, a kind of prefabricated linguistic expression that destroys knowledge instead of increasing it. Memory work is a kind of school of language, an opportunity to try out, to seek out, and to discover words to describe one's own experiences.

Custody

Let us turn to an analysis of the given scene above.

In 1948, shortly after the Second World War, order was far from being restored. Travel possibilities were very inadequate. That forced people to adopt unconventional methods, such as bicycle rides at midnight with children who should have long since been in bed, as indeed their brothers were already. The author describes this as a welcome adventure that gives her added importance as an individual, makes her seem valuable and even indispensable, and credits her with other abilities. Such a position means that she does not just stride out into the hitherto forbidden world of the night; she also estimates her rank of relative insignificance in the hierarchy of the siblings. After all, unlike her brothers, she can carry out a plan, even if it is one her older sister has worked out with her mother. The world of order is left behind; she grows up.

Unlike the scenes with older girls or women, the danger here does not manifest itself initially as a subjective feeling but as a perception on the part of her mother, more or less as a kind of infectious uneasiness. The author also conveys this linguistically: She is not threatened by the darkness or strangeness but rather by "a few drunks wandering around" who "pestered" the family group. Nothing indicates that "drunken" and "pestered" meant anything particular to the author.

Indeed, the fact that her mother sends them away quickly seems at first to be a continuation of the adventure; racing off on the bicycle seems as if it were part of the game.

However, the newly constructed collective "we" of the action soon gives way to the isolated "I" that is pursued by danger. The body begins to speak to her: danger is "pressing in" on them, her eyes signal "lights," she hears "voices," "panting." When the men pass by as she hides in the ditch, she can imagine what danger awaits her. Oddly enough, the original hierarchy has reinstated itself: the men are "after" her sister because she was still "too small." In this way, the growing girl's fear of men is not extinguished—on the contrary, she is out of her mind with fear, but it is explained as a part of growing up. In contrast, she soon learns that you must enlist the protection of the men you know. The bigger you become, the more important this is.

At the same time, the little girl's anxiety is immediately comprehensible. She mobilizes paternalistic feelings, including resentment toward her mother, who sends her daughters "home" under such conditions. However, empathy can do no more than convey the insight that children—especially female ones—should not be allowed out on the streets after dark, mainly when drunk men, not in control of their senses, are out and about. From an analytic standpoint, we discover more about how the ideas of men enter the feminine imagination. While they appear self-explanatory, further questions serve no purpose and seem to call for associating anxiety with men (that is, men are just beings to escape from). On the one hand, these ideas are formed through emotional infectiousness: the mother is afraid, whereas the daughter only sees an adventure. However, the mother represents order, so her violation of customary behavior—which promised to take new significance, usefulness, and growing up—was simultaneously transmitted to the girl as highly problematic. Escape from men is simultaneously a ticket away from her mother. Indeed, it abandoned her to a danger that her mother had drawn attention to. The pursuit of the girls is, in a sense, a liberation from the mother; the privileges bestowed upon the older sister also means an endangerment to them both. In short, the author finds herself in a tangle of contradictory signals that necessarily inhibit any accurate account of, and search for, the real danger.

We come to the following developmental contradictions in the above and other stories: to leave the world of childhood and extend one's ability to act also means trying to escape from the protection and accustomed order of the child's world. The early lesson is that girls need a new protector when they grow out of the old one. Where then, would the satisfaction of growing up lie? However, at the same time, growing up is known to be unavoidable. What additional reserves of curiosity are needed to picture the future dangers men seem to also represent as a supposed source of protection? Can a girl escape from this contradiction simply by ignoring it? Or conversely, what efforts must she make to achieve adulthood in an energetic and self-confident way? How can she live out this inherent contradiction in male images without submitting to them? A preliminary finding seems to be that prefabricated images from various sources can fill the vacant space obscurely occupied by the dangers posed by men. In the above scene, the narrator's perception influences her adventure stories from childhood, in which cops and robbers, hot pursuit, and hide-and-seek games enrich her and our imagination. Such a scene provides a possible way of extending our project into anxiety. We opted for a different route. We examined literature that advises adolescent girls on dealing with such problems. We also referred to fairytales, a cultural building block that impacts our imagination. Here, for example, we discover one solution to the paradox according to which masculinity simultaneously represents threat and protection. Even the examples that appear at first glance as threats only turn into protective beings if you share your table and your bed with them. Men cast off their hedgehog quills or lion skin and slip out of their frog shape only if a woman takes them into her bed.

Sometimes, however, they fail to change and persist as nasty dragons. In such a case, one has to wait for the good man's arrival to provide protection and salvation. In every case, women's activity remains confined to selfless devotion, and the additional piece of advice is: "Do not trust your senses."

Sex and Race

We have seen some of the strange relationships women have with the other sex and with themselves. We also saw how the problem links the perception of nature to society. Both had (and still do have) an impact on the preparedness to discover and obtain knowledge. Character traits that result from this would rather be a tendency to ignore the unknown, avoid communication and interaction, flight, search for protection, and, above all, to never engage with somebody or something strange.

While there is certainly a lot to discover as to the other sex, these other others in our society, there is the additional question of whether this might have any bearing on the issue of strangers in society—that is, the question of racism. I want to present an impression by sharing a final scene, which is also written out of fear for the body by a woman residing in Canada.[8]

Fear for the Body

She said hello to him as she stepped out of the gully beside the park road. She was enjoying the sunshine, mainly the time alone from the rest, as she walked in her shorts and bikini top towards a group she was supposed to visit. She was carrying her T-shirt and a pack of cigarettes. He pointed a gun at her and told her to get down in the gully. Once there, she fell on her knees and begged to be left alone. She thought she would pretend to be hysterical, but soon realized that she was out of control and that probably this was not a good idea, so she tried to rein herself in. He kept pointing off into the jungle and telling her to walk. She kept saying "no." She tried to explain that she was just a Canadian girl who arrived with some kids from school in Santa Marta and was going to visit some of the boys. She said she would not tell anyone if he just let her go. She offered him all she had—her T-shirt and cigarettes. She thought she would pretend she thought he wanted to rob, not rape, her despite him saying, "I just want to be with you."

He would look interested in what she was saying for a few minutes, then say, "Walk." Sometimes, he offered to let her walk in different directions into the jungle as if that would make a difference. She imagined herself spending days/months/years living in the jungle with no water and little food, the prisoner and sex slave of this guy. His hair looked like it had seen neither water nor comb in

> *years—it was all matted together and stuck out all over. He was skinny; his eyes looked a bit crazy. However, she was also afraid of the jungle, knowing she did not know enough to survive alone, so she was not sure running away would be a good idea either. She imagined people wondering forever what had happened to her. Some people went by with a horse and cart. She thought they must have heard them there, but they went by. She thought it was part of his plot.*
>
> *After what seemed like forever but was probably ten minutes, he put away his gun (she does not remember where he put it) and, got out a knife and placed it against her breast. She tried not to flinch. He got angry and yanked her to her feet, saying, "Walk—you can go that way or another way, but walk." She remembered learning to break holds in self-defense class and broke his grasp, scrambling up the ditch to the road and running. She did not think he would shoot her; instead, she thought he might miss because he was too weak and that it was preferable to other options.... He followed her to the road, making the sound Colombian men make when trying to attract a woman's attention. She thought this was nuts but kept running. She flagged down a car full of men. She was afraid of them but more afraid of the guy with the gun.*

Like in all scenes, the author immediately convinces her readers of the danger she is in, the evil coming from the man, and the courage, resistance, and actions she took. The roles are justly distributed: the lovely and friendly innocent western girl against the unfriendly, violent, and dangerous male—who, in this case, is also an inhabitant of someplace near the jungle. Strangely enough, she only told us much later that he was a man of color, though everyone in our group thought so immediately. It was hinted at, although not explicitly said, that this fact structures the whole situation. Let us first look at the description of this guy. He is depicted as dangerous and unpredictable and at the same time as dirty, disgusting, and crazy. He does not wash or comb his hair; he is thin and weak. Whereas she is a Canadian girl who is strong and rational, she can manage even her hysteria; she enjoys the sunshine. She is stronger than he is. At the same time, the scene lives on racism and sexism. It is on the rails of gender relations that she is more afraid of being raped than being shot—though the gun is directed toward her head. She imagines becoming his sex slave for years, unable to escape, stuck with the guy. She has hardly any strategies to escape this spell. In the scene, the decisive point is an empty spot. How does she follow him into the gully if she perceives the gun as not her main threat? Why does she leave the sunshine only to be together with this dangerous man? The author says: "He told her to get down in the gully," and the following words are, "walk over there...." The rationality she tries to develop comes from the superiority of white men.

She insists on being Canadian and from a particular school. She promises not to tell anyone. She offers cigarettes and her T-shirt. All these actions and remarks must sound ridiculous if they were not embedded in a structure where the telling, the offerings, and the nationality meant superiority. At the same time, the man was not supposed to act like he did because he was from a lower kind of people—he was Columbian.

Racism and sexism melt into each other—the man makes the sound "Columbian men make when trying to attract a woman's attention." This is at the same time ridiculous because he was threatening her with a gun only minutes before, rendering Columbian male flirtatious manners into possible violence. Because she is experiencing the whole scene on the foil of gender relations, she would rather die than be raped. Here is the strong woman; all she can think of is offering him her cigarettes and pretending to be hysterical. He is holding a gun between her eyes, but she is not afraid of being shot; she is afraid of being raped. Rape is skimmed over: unspeakable, unthinkable. She thinks rationalizing is her way out of this situation, but the thought of rape terrifies her toward immobilization; in the end, it is not intellect but physical strength that frees her; being unable to go near the thought of rape keeps her from her body, but her body is her power. The strange thing about her story is that the idea of her intellectual superiority, as part of her being white and not Columbian, does not help her in gender relations.

The second strange and notable idea is that she is walking half-naked (in a bikini) in a culture where people walk fully dressed, and this does not even enter her considerations. The lesson we can learn is that women do not have the power in society to manage male violence, but they think they must. The assumption is that male violence is everywhere, but it is more unpredictable the lower the men are in intellect, class, and culture. Somehow, male "nature" and the "nature" of the jungle work together; they are both dangerous. In addition, she feels as if the whole thing "were a plot."

A Conspiracy of Columbians against a White Woman

We have seen this construction of men as bare nature already in gender relations with white men. The only weapon women have is to seek protection through a man of their own. This is useless in confrontation with people of color who are not only perceived as being even closer to a violent "nature" but who are at the same time not seen as possible companions for protection. Whole families are perceived as a male threat and conspiracy. They seem to want to rape white women as a sort of revenge for the whole white colonial culture.

In this situation, the proposition that white superiority reigns over "inferior" men of color is incredibly useless because, for women, it merely implies a superiority of intellect, not of the body. Women are in such a situation precisely because they are women. There is no way to be a woman and survive. Allow me to add one summarizing remark to this first glance at the possibility of using memory work for studies of racism by linking it to studies of sexism. If people perceive each other as sub-human, as possessing violent natures, the whole project of multicultural peace and harmony is no more than an illusion. However, this very perception is part of gender relations. It positions women as always afraid of men because of their "nature" but also in fear for their own "nature." Similarly, men perceive women as being in the order of "nature," even in a different context. The superiority of whites over other ethnic groups is one of the pillars in the perception of others as being less cultural, less intellectual, and more closely tied to nature, which implies being less human. This very pillar and perception remains strong as long as gender relations nourish and guarantee the eternal image of the other sex as being less human than one's own.

The Wicked Uncle

Let us take a step back to girls of pre-school age. A further way of overcoming the contradiction of paradoxical masculinity is the introduction of the "wicked uncle." We assume that the efforts of parents and teachers to create a mysterious aura of unnamed sexuality around men with sweets and, hence, to stop girls from being too trustful toward strange men do not really help girls survive but instead lead to anxiety and an inability to act. This lesson about the "wicked uncle" still occupies a place in the curriculum of the first years at school, even though the threat of sexual abuse is far more likely to come from a trusted member of the family than from strangers in the street.

Understandably, one of our scenes portrays this as the author's chief problem: "What would her parents say if she accepted presents from strange men?" She throws her chocolate bunnies away because she finds even her parents' questions "unpleasant" and "they should on no account learn that the uncle had picked her up and carried her." The event crystallizes in her mind into a kind of crime that is her fault—she is afraid that "everything might come out." Such a scene provides fertile soil for the guides that warn against strange uncles. It is possible to train modes of perception that result in insulating people from the world through fear.

The lesson is that it is dangerous to become involved with the unknown. This attitude is inscribed in relations between the sexes. The contradiction about the wicked uncle described by our author lies in her relationship with such men, in her parents' injunction to beware of strange men. In order to recognize the uncle as a threat, she must be close to him. However, this is the danger her parents warned her to avoid. She incurs guilt if she informs herself. Her chosen strategy of perceiving the uncle's actions as threatening is a violation of their warnings. The contradiction is that she should avoid meeting with any possible evil but must encounter it to recognize it for what it is. The solution can only lie in an early warning system that springs into action long before any danger comes onto the scene.

Preliminary Conclusion

We have thus far achieved preliminary insight into a highly contradictory process of socialization, which, in practice, recommends a retreat into self-denial, domesticity, and submission at every stage of the growing-up process. Contradictions block the path of development and place taboos on the world in an almost archaic manner. They begin with the twofold riddle that men—having been endowed with sexuality long before sexuality has become a real issue—oscillate between familiarity and an alienness that cannot be interrogated. It is inappropriate to explore the badness that is thus intimated. This mindset persists and propagates itself in the world. The world is so harmful and dangerous that a girl should not venture into it, and a woman would be well-advised to stay home. The following contradiction concerns adulthood as such. The desire for liberation, the wish to escape from parental protection, is frustrated by the insight that this can only be achieved at the cost of new protective custody. We thus find that women in a sexual relationship with men are caught up in a contradictory identity, in the sense that they cannot develop their personality without losing it.

The desire for spaces controlled by one's own man is self-denial in the cloak of freedom. There is no experience to which women can appeal that would enable them to find their way around a world they have appropriated in theory without anxiety. Indeed, their knowledge of the world's wickedness stands menacingly in their way, preventing them from setting foot in it.

For our initial question about anxiety in sexual relations and its paradigmatic power in our society, we learned that anxiety about the body is unrestricted to the process of reproduction and women's role in it. On the contrary, the subjugation of the female sex to this social function seems to press both women's bodies and the mysterious male figures into service. Women's acceptance of modesty and retreat, their loss of curiosity and adventurousness, and their renunciation of inquiry and knowledge seem to have been purchased by this anxiety about their bodies, with the consequence that physical anxiety becomes the synthesis of all these experiences. At the same time, it becomes impossible for women to obtain any understanding of these relationships. How can one want to learn about dangers when knowledge itself seems to be a danger?

Curiously, in almost every scene, other women stand as guards blocking the entrance into the world of knowledge and autonomous action. They include sisters, girlfriends, and strangers. Moreover, nowhere do they join forces in search of solutions, nor do they enable them to recognize obstructive contradictions together or discover new modes of acting and living. On the contrary, the danger perceived as coming from men drives women to men for protection. This complexity of danger ensures that heterosexual relationships develop in a way that entails the renunciation of any development at all. We have repeatedly found this strange connection between women's anxieties and the fear of knowledge in widely differing contexts and at different ages and social positions. When we read Christa Wolf's story, *Störfall*,[9] about the nuclear accident at Chernobyl, we found the exact link between anxiety and the fear of knowledge.[10] It seemed important enough to us to warrant making further research into the relationship a significant priority for development. This goes along with the worldwide practice of leaving public affairs to men insofar as they are conducted. Anxiety prevents women from preserving the defeat of the female sex, bringing further anxiety in its wake.

Thus, anxiety makes a double appearance at a strategically significant point; it is both the sign of awakening and the guardian of the different points at which women (as individuals) might break out of the framework to which society assigns them. It is the emotion that both signals an awakening while also impeding and retracting it. This is a vicious circle that we must break.

Notes

1 Editors' Note: This text is part of a larger project on which Frigga Haug worked together with Kornelia Hauser. See Frigga Haug and Kornelia Hauser, ed., *Die andere Angst* (Argument-Verlag, 1991).

2 For a discussion of this, see the Appendix in "The Term 'Angst' and its English Translation," *The Standard Edition of the Complete Psychological Works of Sigmund Freud,* ed. James Strachey, Vol. 3 (Hogarth Press, 1962), 116–117.

3 Brüder Grimm, "Von einem, der auszog, das Fürchten zu lernen," *Kinder- und Hausmärchen,* ed. Heinz Rölleke (Reclam, 1980), 41–49; Jacob Grimm and Wilhelm Grimm, "The Boy Who Set Out to Learn What Fear Was," *The Original Folk and Fairy Tales of the Brothers Grimm,* trans. and ed. Jack Zipes (Princeton University Press, 2014), 20–26.

4 See Sigmund Freud and Josef Breuer, *Studien über Hysterie* (Franz Deuticke, 1895); Sigmund Freud and Josef Breuer, *Studies on Hysteria,* trans. and ed. James Strachey, *The Standard Edition of the Complete Psychological Works of Sigmund Freud,* Vol. 2 (Hogarth Press, 1955). See also Sigmund Freud, *Drei Abhandlungen zur Sexualtheorie* (Franz Deuticke, 1905); Sigmund Freud, *Three Essays on the Theory of Sexuality,* trans. and ed. James Strachey, *The Standard Edition of the Complete Psychological Works of Sigmund Freud,* Vol. 7 (Hogarth Press, 1953).

5 Margaret Atwood has used this syndrome in one of her novels. The main character stays in the forest, expecting that she will gradually grow the fur that will enable her to survive in the wild. Margaret Atwood, *Surfacing* (Bloomsbury, 1972).

6 The term refers to a school that emerged from the work of Aleksei N. Leontiev, Lucien Sève, and Karl Marx, aiming to establish psychology on materialist foundations. Its principal representative was Klaus Holzkamp, who passed away in 1995. Critical Psychology has been active for nearly three decades, producing numerous publications and maintaining its own journal, *Forum Kritische Psychologie*. A defining characteristic of this approach is its historical and developmental method: by tracing the evolution of living beings, it seeks to identify the social as the distinctive feature of humanity and, on this basis, to reconstruct psychology as a whole.

7 Quotation phrases borrowed from *Critical Psychology*, see Note above.

8 Translator's Note: Frigga Haug spent a term as a visiting professor at the Ontario Institute for Studies in Education [OISE], which is linked to the University of Toronto.

9 Christa Wolf, *Störfall. Nachrichten eines Tages* (Luchterhand, 1987).

10 Translator's Note: Christa Wolf was an East German socialist, novelist and essayist who was opposed to German reunification. Employing 'illness' as an ongoing metaphor, her writings explore themes of fascism, feminism and questions of humanity. In her fiction account, Christa Wolf, *Accident: A Day's News,* trans. Heike Schwarzbauer and Rick Takvorian (Farrar, Straus and Giroux, 1989) the protagonist's brother is undergoing surgery to remove a brain tumour following the Chernobyl nuclear disaster.

References

Atwood, Margaret. *Surfacing*. McClelland & Stewart, 1972.

Freud, Sigmund. *Drei Abhandlungen zur Sexualtheorie*. Franz Deuticke, 1905.

Freud, Sigmund. *Three Essays on the Theory of Sexuality*. Translated and edited by James Strachey. *The Standard Edition of the Complete Psychological Works of Sigmund Freud*, Volume 7. Hogarth Press, 1953.

Freud, Sigmund, and Josef Breuer. *Studien über Hysterie*. Franz Deuticke, 1895.

Freud, Sigmund, and Josef Breuer. *Studies on Hysteria*. Translated and edited by James Strachey. *The Standard Edition of the Complete Psychological Works of Sigmund Freud*, Volume 2. Hogarth Press, 1955.

Grimm, Brüder. "Von einem, der auszog, das Fürchten zu lernen." In *Kinder- und Hausmärchen*. Edited by Heinz Rölleke. Reclam, 1980.

Grimm, Brüder. "The Boy Who Set Out to Learn What Fear Was." In *The Original Folk and Fairy Tales of the Brothers Grimm*. Translated and edited by Jack Zipes. Princeton University Press, 2014.

Haug, Frigga, and Kornelia Hauser, eds. *Die andere Angst*. Argument-Verlag, 1991.

Strachey, James. "The Term 'Angst' and its English Translation." In *The Standard Edition of the Complete Psychological Works of Sigmund Freud*. Edited by James Strachey, Volume 3. Hogarth Press, 1962.

Wolf, Christa. *Störfall. Nachrichten eines Tages*. Luchterhand, 1987.

Wolf, Christa. *Accident: A Day's News*. Translated by Heike Schwarzbauer and Rick Takvorian. Farrar, Straus and Giroux, 1989.

Chapter 2

Methodological Questions in Everyday Feminist Research[1]

Frigga Haug

Preliminary Remarks

In the following, I examine questions related to specific feminist approaches to empirical methods. This perspective allows me to bypass the conventional dispute about deconstruction and postmodernism in feminism. During my analysis, I foreground the explanatory and productive aspects of each concept and theoretical orientation. Their relationship to one another, as well as their arrangements for meaningful, liberating feminist knowledge and methodology, are reconstructed in a more critical yet solidarity-based discussion. By no means do I assume that disputes over concepts are ever pointless. On the contrary, it seems to me that the time has come to learn from the various one-sidednesses, criticisms, and errors in a way that transcends them. I offer three proposals for a feminist methodology that differ in their theoretical assumptions and, therefore, yield different conclusions, none of which can claim exclusive representation, but each of which is committed to liberation. This presentation and analysis take place against the background of "general" everyday research. Precisely because I aim to highlight the specificity and productivity of feminist approaches, I present traditional and Marxist everyday research more extensively than is usually the case in feminist contexts. In my opinion, it is necessary to apply feminist critique to the best representatives of "general" sciences, to take them seriously, to build on their strengths, and to transform them by incorporating the feminist standpoint. I first discussed concepts related to women's oppression and their implications for theory and empirical research. Given that all previous science can be considered "male," empirical methods must also be reconstructed. I discuss everyday life as a problem in Marxism and ethnomethodology and then, in contrast, work with feminist methods in their respective specificities. This approach enables me not so much to pit the different feminisms against each other as to demonstrate their feminist-political intervention in the conventional academic world.

Concept Formation and Its Methodological Consequences: In Search of Everyday Life

Feminism has one political option: it is oriented toward women's liberation. In this context of women's liberation, there are several tried and tested concepts—inequality, women's oppression, women's subjugation—that regulate

DOI: 10.4324/9781003480143-2

methodological approaches as well as political practice in ways that are rarely critically reflected upon. If we talk about gender inequality in order to demand equal opportunities, positions, etc., we use quantitative methods with which we count how often and to what extent equality is missed. The figures, statistics, and tables created in this way are certainly necessary material for political practice; however, they do not disrupt conventional scientific production. They adopt its methods and further contribute similar information to the body of knowledge. Such women's studies can be easily incorporated into individual disciplines as a special section.

As a first thesis, I formulate the following: as necessary as the collection of data and facts about the situation of women is, women's studies that limit themselves to this approach will be unable to truly understand the existence of women, make it understandable, and intervene. Presumably, therefore, the concept of inequality is not sufficient. In fact, the accumulation of data on women's unemployment, income, marital status, the proportion of housework performed, the percentage of female university graduates, and so on, has the peculiar effect of remaining external to real-existing women even when they are directly affected. In discussions with women and in their biographical narratives, one easily notices that the collection of data that is immediately important to everyone, such as the average woman's income, is almost always heard as if one does not pertain to oneself, as if one can escape, as if it is someone else's problem—the subjective reasons for escaping are manifold and worthy of investigation in their own right. It is as if classificatory concepts have taken on a life of their own, with meanings that extend beyond the lives of women whose experiences are calling to be recognized differently.

This becomes even clearer in the upheavals and radical shifts caused by the unification of the two Germanies, particularly as the experiences and realities of women from the five new federal states are still unfamiliar to our sociological approach. Yes, even the most familiar concepts, which appear so well-established that a more precise definition of their meaning seems superfluous, elude simple understanding in an uncanny way. Let me offer an example of how the concept of the "family" is assessed by a "Western" and an "Eastern" sociologist (who now resides in England). Ilona Ostner writes:

> Totalitarian, conformist societies are characterised by a lack of differentiation in their social structure: by the lack of subsystems with their own logic that each fulfil specific functions about the respective society. So, marriage and family were also missing. People got married, children were born and lived with their mother and partner(s). However, marriage and family were functionless in a sociological sense.[2]

Peggy Watson writes about the same institution (the family) under the same circumstances (countries of former state socialism):

> In the neo-traditionalist society of Eastern Europe, the family/household, the personal and the private are of central importance… The family is the source of autonomy, an autonomy that is defined not in terms of the claims of the

> individual but in contrast to the state. Although there is a formal and spatial separation between the public and private areas, these areas are, in fact, not comparable to those of the free market economy.[3]

The opposing assessments are based on opposing experiences. The uncritical imposition of concepts onto the uncomprehended bridges the vast area of the unknown and allows it to disappear unrecognized in history. Thus, following the unification, both parts of Germany urgently sought to find common ground in the understanding of the oppression of women and tentatively accomplished this through the concept of the "double burden" on women, which was said to prevail everywhere. Meticulous time calculations lead sociologist Christina Klenner, for example, to the following conclusion: "Women work an average of 4 hours 41 minutes per day in the reproductive sphere (that's domestic work and time for childcare and nursing)...men, on the other hand, only 2.38 hours."[4] It is further calculated that men work an average of 1.18 hours longer, while women have almost an hour less free time. It is certainly helpful to carefully study time consumption; however, it seems to me that the evidence that this constitutes a double burden afflicting women in both the West and the East is surprisingly limited. Should we really assume that in two hours a day (or in one) patriarchy asserts itself existentially and comprehensively? Certainly, such attempts to apply accepted concepts fundamental to Western women's studies to the past of state socialist countries have the beneficial effect of forcing us to rethink these concepts as well.

I will attempt a second common concept: oppression. The word itself points to the weight borne by women and seems to recommend its removal to (as it said) "make women visible," underneath, audible, and public.[5] Methodologically, it entails re-reading, re-discovering women in history, literature, science, and so on, inscribing their deeds in the official history of our societies, and sociologically, it involves procedures that inscribe the "voice" of women into the existing scientific canon. The questions opened up by such conceptual metaphors inevitably struggle with essentialist presuppositions. Previous scientific methods and analyses do not remain entirely unscathed. After all, it is thanks to their arrangements and perspectives that women remain invisible, a blind spot. However, it is largely possible to work within the conventional scientific canon, merely shifting the emphasis.[6]

The third concept I now prefer, female subjugation, opens up a different dynamic space. Agents, circumstances, and a new battlefield come into view. Here, the context is society as a whole, including the sciences and their methods. The "suspicion" that what has hitherto been universal has the gender of the victors of history, and hence the gendering of science as well, critiques methods, concepts, and theories. Reason itself, insofar as it determines our thinking and our ideas about life, is suspected of being a male construction. The liberation of "science" from male one-sidedness and, therefore, from power relations and domination, requires comprehensive destruction and corresponding reconstruction of all previously standard procedures. In this context, I would like to present some attempts to restructure science. I will concentrate here on one area: empirical methods and theoretical considerations for obtaining knowledge about women's socialization processes. At the same time, I examine how far conventional scientific methods have come in this area, their possibilities, and limitations.

On the Problem of Everyday Life: Ethnomethodology and Marxism

It took the political women's movement to discover, even in the university sector, that conventional theories were, and are, conceived without the inclusion of women—not only as creators of theory but also as its objects. The prevailing theories concluded that they do not have to take women's experiences into account. This discovery directs our attention to the space in which experiences are made, a space that, although not fully conceptualized, is immediately understandable: "everyday life." In fact, this critique from the women's movement emerged around the same time as the general shift of some scientific disciplines toward what is considered everyday life.

Since around the mid-70s, the turn to everyday life has become fashionable,[7] but at once, it has been linked from the outset to a critique of conventional social science research—it advocates a turn to the trivial and thus critiques other research for not to taking people's lives seriously. Something peculiar happens here: because everyday events are highlighted as something other than what sociology has done up to now and given a special label (trivial), they are at the same time made exotic. For Alfred Schütz, the father of phenomenological sociology, "The everyday life-world is the region of reality in which man can engage himself and which he can change...."[8] One can see that turning to everyday life is also an admission that "human beings" cannot change the world on a large scale. What is largely missing in the long debates about everyday life as a possible object of science is the mediation between everyday actions and society at large. This means, among other things, that theories (and rules) tend to be sought about everyday life itself and not about how society reproduces itself on a daily basis. The focus was on the study of working conditions, living conditions, everyday culture, and, finally, everyday knowledge. Everyday life as a subject of ethnosociology and methodology is a kind of research field or area that, although cutting across the usual logic of sociology—everyday life is present in industry, in the family, in school, and so on—has its own logic, which can be observed from the outside and whose order can be determined. The consequences of the turn to everyday life for methodological procedures were that the curriculum vitae, the biography, the narrative, and their structures, as well as media analysis, were incorporated into observation and interviews.

A much earlier approach to everyday life comes from Marxist thinking, originating with Marx himself. In "The German Ideology," Marx outlines his research program with repeated reference to the "language of real life," the "real life-process" of human beings, the "real living individuals" "men in the flesh":[9]

> This manner of approach is not devoid of premises. It starts out from the real premises and does not abandon them for a moment. Its premises are men, not in any fantastic isolation and fixity, but in their actual, empirically perceptible

> process of development under definite conditions. As soon as this active life-process is described, history ceases to be a collection of dead facts, as it is with the empiricists (themselves still abstract), or an imagined activity of imagined subjects, as with the idealists...[10]

Marx emphatically emphasizes: "Where speculation ends, where real life starts, there consequently begins real, positive science, the expounding of the practical activity, of the practical process of development of men."[11] The works of Marx and Engels contain numerous studies on everyday life—on housing, nutrition, wood theft, alcohol, etc.; in the official philosophies that crystallized as Marxism or ML (Marxism-Leninism), the main tenet that remained from this context was that being determines consciousness. However, this was not seen as a turn to the study of real "being" and "consciousness" in everyday life, but rather as a form of censorship for empirical research, which keeps under wraps anything that reflects something other than the officially claimed "socialist way of life"—such as alcoholism, rebellious youth cultures, and longing for jeans, etc.

Like erratic signs, demands from Rosa Luxemburg, for example, to write historical research as the work of active everyday people, are reminiscent of Marx's plea quoted above:

> The entire human culture is a work of the social interaction of many, is a work of the masses.... This history (of humanity) is full of heroic legends, of great deeds of individuals, it echoes with the glory of wise kings, bold generals, daring explorers, brilliant inventors, heroic liberators. But all this colorful and beautiful activity of individuals is, so to speak, only the outer floral dress of human history. At first glance, everything good and evil, the happiness and the misery of peoples, is the work of individual rulers or great men. In reality, the people, the nameless masses themselves, make their fate, happiness, and woe.[12]

"No, the pyramids are actually the work of thousands and thousands of patient slaves who, through hard forced labour and moaning loudly, built the stone evidence of their own enslavement."[13] Accordingly, Luxemburg formulated a revolutionary realpolitik that, among other things, takes people's everyday experiences as its starting point, highlights the contradictions they experience as such, and makes them available for those affected to deal with.

Brecht takes up her pictorial suggestions in "Questions from a Worker Who Reads": "Who built Thebes of the seven gates? In the books you will find the names of kings. Did the kings haul up the lumps of rock?... Where, the evening that the Wall of China was finished Did the masons go?"[14]

In a play project dedicated to Rosa Luxemburg, which he titled "Conversation about Everyday Struggle,"[15] the choice between pure abstractions, such as those produced by mathematics, which Luxemburg initially studied, and engagement with everyday life becomes a defining leitmotif. During this period, Brecht wrote about "everyday theatre" as a new task:

You artists who perform plays
In great houses under electric suns
Before the hushed crowd, pay a visit some time
To that theatre whose setting is the street.
The everyday, thousandfold, fameless
But vivid, earthly theatre fed by the daily human contact
which takes place in the street.[16]

The critique is directed at historiography from above. What distinguishes it from the oral history that later became widespread in the 1970s, however, is that it conceives of history itself as the product of the masses, rather than treating the actions of everyday people as something interesting in themselves but taking place outside the actual grand history.

Jürgen Kuczynski extends the criticism of historiography from above to Marxist historiography:

> It is also so often not taken into account that there are, so to speak, two types of class struggles: the big battles and the everyday struggle. Our Marxist historiography basically concentrates on the big battles....But there is hardly anything to be found in our history books about the daily class struggle, whether it be through reluctant work and minor destruction of individual means of production by slaves, or through relatively reduced productivity when performing feudal labor duties compared to working on one's "own" field.[17]

Writing about such things is his project. A further explicit turn to everyday life for research and demonstration purposes as a critical social science program can be found on the side streets of Marxist theory, from the experiences of fascism and Stalinism as early as the 1930s and 1940s; that is, as a correction, as anti-economism, as seen, for example, in Antonio Gramsci and Henri Lefebvre. Gramsci's starting point was the fragmentation of everyday understanding in a contradictory society. From his project of a philosophy of practice, research guidelines for critical empiricism of everyday life can be deciphered: one is a conformist of some kind of conformism, one is always a mass-human or a collective-human. The question is: what historical type is the conformism, the mass-human, in which one participates? If one's view of the world is not critical and coherent, but random and incoherent, one simultaneously belongs to a multitude of mass people, and one's personality is bizarrely composed: it contains elements of the caveman and principles of the most modern and advanced science, prejudices of all past, locally narrow-minded historical phases and intuitions of a future philosophy that will be united by a globally united human race. To critique one's own worldview means to make it unified and coherent and to raise it to the point reached by the most advanced thinking in the world. It, therefore, also means critiquing the entire previous philosophy insofar as it has left behind entrenched stratifications in popular philosophy. The beginning of critical elaboration is what is real, that is, "know thyself" as a product of the historical process that has taken place thus far, which has left an infinity of traces within yourself, an inventory of your legacy accepted without reservation. Such an inventory must be created at the outset.[18] "Real people" can, therefore, act in intellectual submission and subordination and yet, at the same time, follow a different practice; in short, their common sense is contradictory. They harbor at least "two theoretical consciousnesses": one derived from the practice that determines them, and another which they have uncritically adopted from the past. In this way, individuals reach the point "where the contradiction of consciousness does not allow any action, any decision, any choice, and produces a state of moral and political passivity."[19] It is necessary for individuals to work their way out of such unlivable disintegration and incoherence and to become self-aware and thus capable of action. Gramsci calls this "giving one's actions a conscious direction." To do this, they must become, as he calls them, "philosophers." For him, this means achieving a coherent worldview with which they can agree. The only way to do this is through a joint social project aimed at social change. This is because the problem of their being torn apart from behind is also a result of the fact that individuals are not involved in the social projects or are involved in a subjugated form. Such a circumstance, in turn, creates the need for so-called "organic intellectuals" in this project, who pave the way for everyone to be an intellectual. Their task is not to "introduce a science into everyone's individual life" but rather to renew an already existing activity in order to make it "critical."[20]

Without referring to Gramsci, Henri Lefebvre comes to very similar conclusions.

> The consciousness of the work involves—together with the content of his own practical experience—numerous ideological elements, some justified, others illusory; some atavistic (coming, for example, from the peasant or artisan classes); others deriving from objective but partly outmoded conditions of capitalism (the 'free' labour contract in competitive capitalism, the 'classic' forms of class struggle); still others derived from the new conditions within capitalism (monopolies, new content contradicting the monopolistic form of capitalism; trade union action and new forms of class struggle); others deriving from socialism, and finally others coming from individual limits or the limits of the group the worker in question belongs to (corporatism, professional solidarity, etc.) social practices as a whole, to his experience as a whole, his leisure activities, his family life, his cultural and political goals, as well as to the class struggle. What is more, this 'whole' must be taken in the context of a specific country and nation, at a specific moment of civilization and social development, and as involving a certain set of needs. And this brings us back to the critique of everyday life.[21]

Lefebvre's project was—quite analogous to the critique of political economy—to write a critique of everyday life, which he understood as a contradictory movement, as a place of the movement of alienation and as a struggle against it.[22] In the middle of the text, he says in capital letters: "*THUS MARXISM, AS A WHOLE, REALLY IS*

A CRITICAL KNOWLEDGE OF EVERYDAY LIFE."[23] His starting point is Marx's project from "The German Ideology." He sees it as a guide for exploring everyday life, uncovering the dormant and twisted forces within it, and using critique as a revolutionary weapon: "Thus the critique of everyday life involves a critique of political life, in that everyday life already contains and constitutes such a critique: in that it is that critique."[24]

Lefebvre's central concepts are alienation and appropriation. He draws both from historical and philosophical uses into everyday life. By critiquing everyday life, he deciphers the division between public and private, indeed private life itself as a common expression of the inversion of everyday life, the role of ideology, its entry into everyday life, and its simultaneous reproduction within it. He carries out media analysis and formulates a general research hypothesis that "everyday life is the place in which and from which the real creations are accomplished, those that produce the human and, in the course of their humanization, people: the deeds and works."[25] Everyday life must, in keeping with Gramsci, be worked through coherently by individuals. Starting from everyday life, knowledge is linked to changing practice, and a theory of social change is linked to a paradigm shift in the sciences. From people's practices, conventional theoretical constructs become decipherable as curious images, ideologies, and speculations. His research leads him to ideology critique as critical media analysis and to the study of alternative films and plays (Chaplin and Brecht). He examines changing technical conditions in households and leisure behavior, among other things. However, his analyses do not lead him to include everyday people in the research framework itself.

Situated between ethnosociology and Marxism, Habermas identifies a break in everyday life when "communicative everyday world is decomposed by systemic structures" when a "systemically induced reification'[26] takes place, and the life world is cut off from 'cultural tradition'."[27] He writes:

> In the deformations of everyday practice, symptoms of rigidification combine with symptoms of desolation. The former, the one-sided rationalization of everyday communication, goes back to the growing autonomy of media-steered subsystems, which not only get objectified into a norm-free reality beyond the horizon of the lifeworld, but whose imperatives also penetrate into the core domains of the lifeworld. The latter, the dying out of vital traditions, goes back to a differentiation of science, morality, and art, which means not only an increasing autonomy of sectors dealt with by experts, but also a splitting-off from traditions; having lost their credibility these traditions continue along on the basis of everyday hermeneutics as a kind of second nature that has lost its force.[28]

Habermas does not assume, like Lefebvre and others, that counter-rationality can be anchored in everyday life, but rather that the prevailing rationality of the system even corrodes everyday life, which we are supposed to imagine as determined by familiarity and understanding.

Feminist Interventions

From a feminist standpoint, a blind spot in all such attempts, however sympathetic they may be, is striking. Without exception, the research design is such that women's lives must become invisible. Whether, as with Habermas, decompositions only occur with the intrusion of the system worlds, instead of seeing lifeworlds and their locations (such as family, privacy, intimacy, and closeness) themselves as battlegrounds, as sites of subjugation, power, and domination; whether, as in Lefebvre's case, the problem is assumed to be exclusively between alienation and liberation from capitalist exploitation, even if everyday life is now comprehensively included in the concept as the site of such a struggle, and not just the workplace; whether, as in the case of Luxemburg and Brecht, the focus is on the producers of capital and the attack is aimed at the historical records of the great names; or whether, finally, one seeks general structures of everyday life and corresponding communicative processes (for example, Garfinkel, Schütz, Luckmann), as if it were not necessary to assume predetermined processes of power and domination or subjugation with corresponding consequences for gender-specific everyday actions as well as methodological procedures. However, Gramsci's intervention extends beyond the other proposals in terms of method, even though it also does not appear sufficient for the inclusion of women's experiences in scientific research and the associated radical methodological changes.

A further turning point in questions of everyday life came about through the women's movement. To proclaim the "personal as political" meant thinking of everyday life as a political battleground, but also as a source from which knowledge can be drawn about the many hidden dimensions of female socialization, the production of femininity, the workings of ideology, power, and domination, and, at the same time, as a field from which reconstructions can be made, including alternative methods of acquiring knowledge.

In what follows, I would like to introduce three feminist projects that, in different ways, represent paradigm shifts for conventional methods of doing sociology or social psychology: Dorothy Smith's project, Carol Gilligan's project, and finally, the project I am working on, memory work.

Sociology for Women—Dorothy Smith's Project[29]

In ethnosociological and methodological considerations—even up to Habermas' ideas about the different rationalities of system and lifeworld—the problem arises again and again that everyday actions and knowledge require the use of different logics, structures, and concepts than those used in the conventional scientific system. What is conceived here as coexistence or mere otherness is reformulated by the Canadian Dorothy Smith as a problem of gender relations and as a general critique of sociological knowledge and the associated systems and concepts. From her experiences in the women's movement and the rapid and groundbreaking learning processes that were possible there, she concludes that the strangeness and emptiness that she experienced as a woman in sociology were not due to her inadequacy, but rather to the absence of women and thus of physical existence in general in the construction of science itself along with its central assumptions and concepts.

From the experience that the conventional sociological concepts do not fit women's lives, actions, and feelings, she does not conclude that new, suitable concepts and theorems should be derived from female experience and, in this way, set up an empirical research project. Instead, she concludes that the dominant systems of science, state bureaucracies, social apparatuses, and bureaucracies not only operate with concepts and systems that exclude women, but that these concepts/systems themselves subsequently regulate society and thereby gain access to women's lives. From the strangeness that sociological theorems represented for her own everyday life, she designs an empirical project that seeks out the refuse between women's general "previous" practical experiences and other experiences they have with the concepts that regulate society and are rooted in sociology, as well as the perceptions determined by these concepts. Her goal is to make the connection between everyday experience and the level of social regulations understandable to those affected by it—in this case, women. The procedure/method itself has a general claim to validity.

The starting point and prerequisite for such a project are three observations and conclusions:

1 The lack of inclusion of female experiences in sociological conceptual language and systems of thought, which for Smith as a sociologist, meant a similar disregard for herself, with all the consequences that this has for scientific imagination and usefulness.
2 The influx of energy that self-consciousness groups in the women's movement also brought to questions of knowledge, without, however, their mediation by higher levels of social regulation being recognizable in such experiences themselves.
3 The questionable nature of science and scientists who do not make their skills and tools available to those they are nevertheless concerned with, and who live, as it were, fatefully in an unrecognized world.

This paradigm shift relates to two dimensions. First, the obligation of scientific processes to make the world understandable as a social production for those who live in it, that is, to contribute to people's ability to act on a daily basis—this concerns the standpoint of scientific work and its connection to a social/political project. Second, a shift in perspective: the subject of their sociological research will be—perhaps to put it in a somewhat exaggerated way—concepts (texts) as powers that intervene in and regulate human lives.

Here I illustrate this procedure using two examples. Recently, several previously private acts have been brought into the public eye: the sexual abuse of children, particularly girls, in addition to the general neglect and abandonment of children; violence against women in marriage (general physical violence as well as rape); and neglect and violence against the elderly. All these acts, which cast the family, that place of intimacy and trust, as an inhospitable space of brutality and domination that had to be publicly remedied, called for a common concept to be found for what was happening here. With the collaboration of feminists, the concept of "domestic violence" was proposed. The concept became material violence. The Ministry of Family Affairs took it up and allocated it, or the department so named, a fund (not a large one, of course). As a result, the various civil initiatives suddenly found themselves as fierce opponents. *The Child Protection Association* fought the claims of feminists who, like *Wildwasser* in this country, focused primarily on the sexual abuse of girls, and both, of course, had to downplay the importance of the abuse of the elderly as a secondary problem. The example should serve to demonstrate that concepts—i.e., abstractions from everyday concreteness—intervene in people's relationships and regulate their practices.

Another empirical project deals with shifts in perception regarding one's own self. Take, for example, instances where mothers in guardianship proceedings learn that they must comment on the concept of "in the best interests of the child," which is intended to regulate which parent the child is better off with (which is at least progress compared to the previously common practice of deciding on the basis of guilt). Questioned in this way, a mother may assume that it is in the child's best interest to tell them a bedtime story, to answer their questions, to be present at all times, or conversely, to allow them to frequently spend time with friends, even to stay overnight away from home, etc. She will have to be taught that income and one's moral lifestyle are decisive and will henceforth be forced to look at and evaluate herself with such eyes, and to consider what she previously thought as unimportant. The intervention goes against one's self-esteem as well as previous experience.

Empirical research starts with a conflict, seeks out the conceptual formulation, and rearticulates the different experiences that are summarized in the concept and from which it abstracts. It shows abstraction as a specific act of power and displacement and the concept as material violence which the original female actors find it difficult to live with. The proposal would have to be a different conceptual and practical strategy.

A central assumption and, at the same time, the result of such research, is the idea of rejection, of rupture, of seeming insignificance, of empowerment. An important field of research is ideology critique; ideology is understood as a strategy of classification and normalization that guarantees, or at least helps, secure and support the functioning of society. In this sense, previous sciences are also ideology, insofar as they help shape and regulate people's experiences but do not actually originate from them. It is understandable that from women's point of view, this project holds special significance.

On the Dissociation of Women: A Proposal by Carol Gilligan[30]

Carol Gilligan gained recognition in Germany for her book *The Other Voice*, in which she critiques Kohlberg's seven stages of moral development as an androcentric construction. She proposes a relationship-oriented and caring ethic for women in opposition to his idea of justice as the highest guiding principle for action. The subsequent discussion, as well as Kohlberg's expansive practice, which enabled him to easily incorporate such a suggestion into his research,[31] prompted her to expand her research framework as a paradigm shift. In her more recent work, she claims that women are fundamentally divided in this society—she refers to it as "dissociated." As adolescents, girls have experiences that society interprets differently from the way they make practical sense of them. During adolescence, they must decide whether they "want to know" or be "accepted" as belonging. Or, to put it another way: socially accepted ideas of a good woman, a good girl, a good mother, a good relationship, and so on, do not correspond to their own insights into social contexts. As a result, they end up in a state where they do not (want to) know what they know. Or, in other words, they must give up their personality in order to keep it. In such paradoxes, they "dissociate" from themselves. So much from the theoretical assumptions. Methodologically, Gilligan follows an approach that we might perhaps describe as "track reading." She looks for that dissociation and its description in women's literature. She conducts conversations with adolescent girls on the specific question of how knowledge is unlearned and replaced by ignorance, and how this is also quantitatively reflected in the language, as evidenced by the rapidly growing number of "I do not know" statements interspersed throughout answers, which, as the situation becomes more familiar, alternate with "You know," and so on. The project aims to strengthen the level of social classification of previous experiences and social perception; it is, therefore, also a social project of liberation, with its starting point being the alienation of women in our societies. Kohlberg's framework of continuous advancement in moral development, with simultaneous integration into society, is thus abandoned. Gilligan's message is that women cannot integrate without losing themselves. Revolt is called for. To achieve this, women must share their experiences and listen to each other in order to reverse their alienation from themselves.

In this process, they will find no support in the dominant social culture. The title of her first book, *The Other Voice*, is strangely oriented in this way. The "other voice" is not the voice of women as opposed to that of men, but rather, in a sense, the second voice that wants to be heard beneath the ordinary, normalized voice of adult women.

Rejection, rupture, division—what feminist interventions have in common is that they assume that under conditions and relations of domination and power, damage is experienced, which makes active efforts to change such living conditions difficult or even impossible. Women are divided, misjudge their knowledge, and fail to recognize the forces that silence them and make them incapable of action. Insofar as it is tied to a liberation project, the interventionist analysis can provide support and enable those who have been silenced to speak. Feminist scholars, therefore, see themselves, as Gramsci would have put it, as organic intellectuals in the women's movement.

It is evident that both Dorothy Smith's ideas for developing a sociology that makes structural connections understandable to women who, for systemic reasons, cannot see them from their position, and Carol Gilligan's premise of the inconsistency, even tornness, of women are compatible with Gramsci's suggestions for dealing with common sense, as presented above. (However, neither one of them was able to read Gramsci's work sufficiently, as the complete English edition of the *Prison Notebooks* is only now being published). A specific distinction and shift arises when it comes to the question of gender relations. Gramsci's idea that it is necessary to achieve a conscious relationship with one's own history and to participate together in the social project of the "social future" is, in turn, based only on *one* relationship of domination. Gramsci expands simple premises about all-determining relations of production to include the idea of an unconsciously non-simultaneous relationship to one's own past, which can only be worked out coherently through social participation. However, there is no room for the problem that, even in such non-simultaneous situations, women's subjugation is part of normality and also unequally affects the project of social participation. The limitations on the possibility, indeed on the desire to acquire knowledge, because the costs are too high, as Carol Gilligan has shown, make a different intervention necessary for women.

Memory Work: On the Connection between Agency and Everyday Research[32]

Based on very similar observations to those presented so far, I, along with others, have also developed a project for women's studies: memory work. The starting point here is also the absence of experience in science—at least as far as women's everyday lives are concerned—and the absence of concepts of experience. The different positioning of women scientists—as people who make the world understandable for the many who live in it—emerged to a certain extent from methodological and theoretical considerations.

So, I did not initially take the path of examining, like Dorothy Smith, these major concepts of sociology—such as state, law, society, economy, interest, organization, and institution—in relation to women's everyday experiences. Instead, I looked the other way around: what is of orienting importance for women in their lives, what areas and phenomena are concentrated in women's everyday lives, and what terminology can capture women's experience and female practices from the bottom up, so to speak. In doing so, I came across well-known phenomena that affect and concern people on an existential level, such as: morality, guilt and fear, the experience of time, happiness, love, power, daydreaming, sexuality, achievement, learning, desire to work, and laziness. The peculiarity of such areas and phenomena is that they can be recognized directly and consensually as essential for social behavior and socialization. Their tense relationship to sociological concepts does not mean that they are too commonplace, so to speak, that they belong therefore in a subsystem of medium-range theory formation. On the contrary, they are theoretically very strong, but, in the division of our scientific disciplines, they have fallen elsewhere—into the personal theories of psychology and psychoanalysis and the wide-ranging realms of philosophy.

We conducted empirical qualitative research with women on the major topics mentioned above, which suddenly led us to a discovery that, albeit always anticipated, was nevertheless peculiar. Even with concepts that clearly affect women directly, the theoretical articulations in philosophy and psychology/psychoanalysis regarding such existential phenomena as morality, guilt, and fear do not include women's experiences and actions, or do so only very speculatively. The concepts are binary, and the proportion of women still needs to be determined in order to be theoretically comprehensible. What is obviously needed here is a different type of theory formation.

This fact makes research work multifaceted. It is no longer just a matter of restructuring sociology or psychology, of crossing scientific boundaries to make women's social actions generally theorizable and understandable to them; it is also about women's experiences themselves being the source of such knowledge, even though they are contradictorily determined. These are experiences in a society in which, both practically and theoretically, women are accorded a place insofar as they are perceived as human beings and, a particular place, insofar as they are women. In short, women in our societies have different experiences that can come into conflict with one another, and each needs to harmonize and balance these experiences in their perception and processing. Orientation is provided by norms and values, socially recognized meanings, which, for women, form a subsystem under the generally accepted orientation system. For example, morality for men primarily relates to politics and business, while for women, it relates to the body and sexuality—yet women also know that it is immoral to forge a check.

The proposal of carrying out memory work also assumes incoherence among the people involved, which is difficult for them to live with. The initial question is that of the sociality of women. One of the theoretical prerequisites is that femininity is a social construction and that becoming a woman is, therefore, a historical and cultural process, the study of which requires knowledge of the structure and organization of society. However, the research question is: How do girls integrate themselves into social structures and thereby transform them so that they can act and find meaning within them?

The way the question is formulated attempts to avoid two problems that we often encounter in empirical research: either thinking of everything as predetermined or determined and derivable from social conditions and accordingly elaborated, or, conversely, placing actions and behaviors too subjectively at the discretion of individuals alone. Instead, the object of investigation is what is perceived by individuals from their circumstances and society, given meaning, and incorporated into their own lives.

Theories do not lead us to female experiences; starting from the latter, however, means making them theoretically accessible, decoding their implementation through ideologies and through external- and self-determination. The only ones who "know" how they have worked their way into society are the affected women themselves. Sociologically speaking, they are the epistemic material. However, since experience does not simply speak for itself and therefore cannot simply be compiled into knowledge, the process is more complicated. It is necessary to investigate how lessons were learned from experiences and how nothing could be learned from other experiences; which paths were chosen as meaningful and assigned subjective significance, and which were rejected; in short, how the social construction of femininity as an ideal target was itself appropriated, transformed, rejected, reproduced, and produced. Trying to decipher the construction of oneself in a critical engagement with society shifts the objects of research—women—into the status of subjects, making them researchers of their own socialization.

The process is more complicated than it sounds. The feminist-methodological postulate of not researching women as if they were insects,[33] but of resolving the subject-object question in favor of joint research, becomes here a postulate of the inner necessity of the process itself. For both movements, making oneself the object and being the subject who conducts research requires competence. In memory work, as one possible way of approaching the problem, we try to undertake a different kind of objectification. It is not women as fragile, incoherent, and "dissociated" personalities who enter the research process, researching themselves or being researched, but instead texts and memory scenes written by them.

A theoretical premise underlying this approach is the view that the past, or rather the way we perceive the past, has significance for actions and behavior in the present and for the way we move forward into the future. We do not assume that the various components are simply lying around in a disordered manner within individual personalities but instead follow Leontiev's[34] view that personality has a memory.[35] This means that the past is not simply stored in memory. Rather, a selection has been made, a set of memory-relevant pieces has been compiled, so to speak, which determines our personalities or constructs our perception of ourselves as a relatively consistent and contradictory person. For example, we can perceive ourselves as failures and have scenes ready to prove this, or conversely as consistently successful, without being unable to "have" both memories at one's disposal. The past, even our own, is therefore not simply available to us as such but is already a construction, a selection, a specific meaning that is important for our personality today.

To examine the historical-cultural development of personality in all its complexity, it is first necessary to distance oneself from experience in the form of the remembered and written text, which, being written as a scene for a specific situation, is, as expected, usually composed of a variety of details and allows several construction methods to be deciphered. Using linguistic and discourse analysis methods, these texts are deconstructed in the group to decipher their construction methods as self-made, as constructions of the self and society, and their subjectively perceived connection. The assumption here—like Gilligan's—is that the different voices emerge in the text from different experiences and social expectations, and that they can be deciphered as contradicting each other, as breaks, as inconsistencies with the overlaid meaning.

Incidentally, this is not simply an unsettling process, as one might assume from the above, but often an enjoyable one, because one can discover oneself in adventurous constructions of plausibility that can never stand up to one's theoretical perspective. The memories, thus, prove to be not only a treasure trove of insights into socialization, but also a mixture of ideologies, everyday theories—that mixture of theoretical bits that have sunk into everyday life and common sense—that contain artful eliminations of contradictions in favor of agency.

This complexity and embeddedness of the experience and construction of memory in society repeatedly repositions the participants involved in a research group. The women in the group, whose social integration is at stake, experience themselves less as fated and thrown, or as having no alternatives in everyday life, but rather as having become autonomous in certain practices, with specific perceptions, meanings, harmonizations, selections, etc. This means that in order not to lose their agency, they must change.

Memory work, therefore, is, or aims at: a critique of practice and critique of social perception; it is also a critique of theory. The scientist—even if there is only one in the research group—is also not spared from change: not only is she herself a subject-object of research—one among many—she is also called upon as a theorist who provides the instruments of deconstruction, who knows the theories that occupy the field, and who drives its critical change. She acts as an "organic intellectual" in Gramsci's sense. She is also challenged by the necessary transgression of disciplinary boundaries—a sacrilege in the conventional scientific canon. Her critique is also directed a second time at sociology. The fact that the central concepts of sociology, when attempted to be learned from a dictionary, cannot be applied to the social experience of women, and that, conversely, existentially essential experiences lead to other sciences like psychology and philosophy, gives rise to the suspicion that sociology may not be an empirical science at all; that sociology's reference to experience is due to its detachment from everyday life, it in itself an artificial disembodied existence, which, if described as experience, has the negation of women's everyday life as one of its foundations, as Dorothy Smith and many other feminist theorists of the critique of reason and rationality claim.

Does such a critique mean that women researchers in sociology must now become philosophers or psychologists? Using a brief example from research on anxiety and its psychoanalytic treatment, I would like to demonstrate that such a choice is not the consequence of this critique but rather that the latter targets the division of disciplines and advocates its transgression—not the abandonment, but instead the expansion of sociological and psychological questions.

Anxiety is certainly a feeling that orients, blocks, renders agency impossible, and determines social relationships. While philosophical considerations generally connect anxiety as a primal feeling with people's mortality, thus asserting the fear of death as a primal anxiety (for example, Kierkegaard[36]), women are often seen as entangled in the anxiety of life. Anxiety orients their steps in public, in darkness, in work, and in time. Freud suggested that such a widespread feeling, as he observed in his female patients, could be linked to a distorted, mass social practice; he later assumed that anxiety arises from a contradiction that individuals cannot resolve on their own. By focusing solely on sexual practices, he inevitably overlooked the fact that all social practices in which women are involved are contradictory, and he also failed to look beyond the internal, beyond the relationship between ego/id/superego, to see the social arrangement itself as contradictory and therefore frightening for women. Feminist science, on the other hand, will not assume that people simply experience society (or the state or economy) nor that their feelings have no significance for social perception, social behavior, and action.

The expansion of the sociological inquiry also makes feminist research, among other things, cultural studies. By culture, or rather by the cultural, I mean—again following Gramsci, Irene Dölling, the CCCS,[37] Wolfgang Fritz Haug, and others—how individuals appropriate society, transform conditions, fill them with life, and find meaning in the process of affirming themselves as human beings. Researching this process sociologically as a historical-cultural one, in my opinion, must begin with the subjects themselves, their experiences in society, and their solutions for their agency. By agency, I mean the ability to influence the conditions of one's own actions.

Individuals and society are thus conceived as historical products, as made history that can be understood and, consequently, also critiqued and changed. Memory work is *one* proposal for how empirical methods could be carried out. It has the advantage of combining the critique of ideology, language, everyday life, theory, society and culture; it has the disadvantage that an organizing scientist, with knowledge of structure and organization, theory and ideology, in as many areas as possible, is necessary for the research work itself and yet, at the same time, must also appear as an equal on the level of experience. This contradiction still needs to be worked through.

* * *

Once, there was a dispute as to whether feminist methods even existed or whether women's studies simply applied well-known and proven methods to women's lives and social situations. To the extent that a decision is even possible in such disputes, it was in favor of methodological neutrality.[38] With this insight into different feminist interventions, I aim to demonstrate, among other things, that a paradigm shift is indeed necessary at all levels. Feminist research is linked to a socio-political project; it starts from contradictions and ruptures; it changes the position of female scientists and that of research "objects"; disciplinary boundaries are almost systematically crossed; the structure and function of sciences are shifted; a variety of methodological approaches alternate with one another, forming, so to speak, a methodological grid or arrangement—the method itself remains always in development. Both social change and self-change are implied. The extent to which the new proposals can later find their way into the general scientific canon remains to be seen. Overall, however, it becomes clear, among other things, that feminist science itself is a civil society project, an attempt to consciously combine one's socialization with knowledge, thereby expanding and advancing it from below.

Notes

1 Editors' Note: A version of this article was published in German as "Alltagsforschung als zivilgesellschaftliches Projekt," *Das Argument,* no. 206 (1994): 639–658.
2 Ilona Ostner, "Die Beschränktheit der Totalen. Anmerkungen einer empirischen Soziologin," *Ethik und Sozialwissenschaften* 4, no. 2 (1993): 252–254.
3 Peggy Watson, "Osteuropa: Die lautlose Revolution der Geschlechterverhältnisse," *Das Argument* 202, no. 6 (1993): 859–874, 869.
4 Christina Klenner, "Doppelt belastet oder einfach ausgebeutet? Zur Aneignung weiblicher Reproduktionsarbeit in DDR-Familien," *Das Argument* 184, no. 6 (1990): 865–874, 867.
5 For feminist critiques of science in its historical development see, for example, Sandra Harding, *Feministische Wissenschaftstheorie. Zum Verhältnis von Wissenschaft und sozialem Geschlecht* (Argument Verlag, 1990).
6 See, for instance, the recent debate on feminist ethics, in which—at least according to some of its female representatives—the male ethicists themselves are identified as authors who also spoke with a female voice. One example among many is Annette C. Baier, "Hume, der Moraltheoretiker der Frauen?," *Jenseits der Geschlechtermoral: Beiträge zur feministischen Ethik,* ed. Herta Nagl-Docekal and Herlinde Pauer-Studer (Suhrkamp, 1993), 105–134; Annette C. Baier, "Hume, the Women's Moral Theorist?," *Women and Moral Theory,* ed. Eva Feder Kittay and Diana T. Meyers (Rowman & Littlefield, 1987), 37–55.
7 See Peter Alheit, *Alltagsleben. Zur Bedeutung eines gesellschaftlichen "Restphänomens"* (Campus, 1983).
8 Alfred Schütz and Thomas Luckmann, *Strukturen der Lebenswelt* (Suhrkamp, 1979), 25; Alfred Schütz and Thomas Luckmann, *The Structures of the Life-World,* trans. Richard M. Zaner and H. Tristram Engelhardt, Jr. (Northwestern University Press, 1973), 3.
9 Karl Marx, "German Ideology," *Marx Engels Werke Band* 3 (Dietz, 1969), 9–439, 26; Karl Marx, "The German Ideology," *Marx and Engels Collected Works, Volume 5: Marx and Engels 1845–47* (International Publishers, 1976), 36.
10 Marx, "German Ideology," 27; Marx, "The German Ideology," 37.
11 Marx, "German Ideology," 27; Marx, "The German Ideology," 37.
12 Rosa Luxemburg, *Gesammelte Werke Band 4: August 1914 bis Januar 1919* (Dietz 2003), 206.
13 Luxemburg, *Gesammelte Werke Band 4,* 207.
14 Bertolt Brecht, "Fragen eines lesenden Arbeiters, " *Gedichte 2, Gesammelte Werke 9* (Suhrkamp, 1967), 656–657; Bertolt Brecht, *Poems Part Two: 1920–1938,* ed. John Willet and Ralph Manhem (Methuen, 1976), 252.

15 Brecht, "Gespräch über den Alltagskampf," *Gedichte 3*, *Gesammelte Werke 10*, (Suhrkamp 1967), 966–967.
16 Brecht, "Gedichte aus dem Messingkauf," *Gedichte 2*, *Werke 12*, ed. Werner Hecht, Jan Knopf, Werner Mittenzwei and Klaus-Detlef Müller (Aufbau Verlag/Suhrkamp Verlag, 1988), 319–331, 319; Brecht, "On Everyday Theatre," *Poems: 1913–1956*, ed. John Willet and Ralph Manheim (Methuen, 1976), 176.
17 Jürgen Kuczynski, *Geschichte des Alltags des deutschen Volkes* (Pahl-Rugenstein, 1981), 13.
18 Antonio Gramsci, "Philosophie der Praxis," *Gefängnishefte*, ed. Klaus Bochmann and Wolfgang Fritz Haug, Vol. 6, Heft 12, §12 (Argument, 1994), 1376; Antonio Gramsci, *Selections from the Prison Notebooks* (International Publishers, 1971), 324.
19 Gramsci, "Philosophie der Praxis," Heft 11, §12, 1384; Gramsci, *Selections from the Prison Notebooks*, 333.
20 Gramsci, "Philosophie der Praxis," Heft 11, §12, 1375.
21 Henri Lefebvre, *Kritik des Alltagslebens*, *Band I* (Athenäum Verlag, 1977), 95–96; Henri Lefebvre, *Critique of Everyday Life* (Verso, 2014), 125–126.
22 See Lefebvre, *Kritik des Alltagslebens*, Bd. II, 77.
23 Lefebvre, *Kritik des Alltagslebens*, Bd. I, 153; Lefebvre, *Critique of Everyday Life*, 148. Editors' Note: In both the original French and the German translation of Lefebvre's *Critique of Everyday Life,* this sentence appears in capital letters, but not in the English version. To preserve the intended meaning of Frigga's sentence, we have amended the English translation and rendered the quote in all capital letters.
24 Lefebvre, *Kritik des Alltagslebens*, Bd. I, 100; Lefebvre, *Critique of Everyday Life*, 130.
25 Lefebvre, *Kritik des Alltagslebens*, Bd. II, 52; Lefebvre, *Critique of Everyday Life*, 339.
26 Jürgen Habermas, *Theorie des kommunikativen Handelns*, *Band 2* (Suhrkamp, 1981), 212, 481; Jürgen Habermas, *The Theory of Communicative Action*, Vol. II, trans. by Thomas McCarthy (Beacon Press, 1987), 277.
27 Habermas, *Theorie des kommunikativen Handelns*, 483; Habermas, *The Theory of Communicative Action*, 277.
28 Habermas, *Theorie des kommunikativen Handelns*, 483; Habermas, *The Theory of Communicative Action*, 278.
29 See Dorothy E. Smith, *The Everyday World as Problematic* (Northeastern University Press, 1987).
30 See Carol Gilligan, *Die andere Stimme. Lebenskonflikte und Moral der Frau* (Piper, 1984); Carol Gilligan, *In a Different Voice. Psychological Theory and Women's Development* (Harvard University Press, 1982).
31 See, among others, Gertrud Nunner-Winkler (ed.), *Weibliche Moral. Die Kontroverse um eine geschlechtsspezifische Ethik* (Suhrkamp, 1991) and *Social Research* 50, no. 3 (Autumn 1983).
32 See Frigga Haug, *Erinnerungsarbeit* (Argument, 1990); Frigga Haug, *Female Sexualization: A Collective Work of Memory* (Verso, 1987).
33 Especially Maria Mies, "Methodische Postulate zur Frauenforschung," *Beiträge zur feministischen Theorie und Praxis*, Heft 1: Erste Orientierungen (Verlag Frauenoffensive, 1978), 41–64.
34 Aleksei Nikolayevich Leontiev, *Probleme der Entwicklung des Psychischen* (Athenäum Fischer Taschenbuch Verlag, 1973).
35 Klaus Holzkamp, *Grundlegung der Psychologie* (Campus, 1983).
36 See for instance Søren Kierkegaard, *The Concept of Anxiety: A Simple Psychologically Orienting Deliberation on the Dogmatic Issue of Hereditary Sin*, trans. Reidar Thomte in collaboration with Albert B. Anderson (Princeton University Press, 1980).

37 Editors' Note: Frigga Haug is referring here to the *Centre for Contemporary Cultural Studies*, a research centre that was founded by Stuart Hall and Richard Hoggart at the University of Birmingham.
38 Reginae Becker-Schmidt, "Frauen und Deklassierung. Geschlecht und Klasse," *Klasse und Geschlecht*, ed. Ursula Beer (AJZ-Verlag, 1987), 187–235.

References

Alheit, Peter. *Alltagsleben. Zur Bedeutung eines gesellschaftlichen "Restphänomens."* Campus, 1983.

Baier, Annette C. "Hume, der Moraltheoretiker der Frauen?" In *Jenseits der Geschlechtermoral: Beiträge zur feministischen Ethik*. Edited by Herta Nagl-Docekal and Herlinde Pauer-Studer. Suhrkamp, 1993.

Baier, Annette C. "Hume, the Women's Moral Theorist?" In *Women and Moral Theory*. Edited by Eva Feder Kittay and Diana T. Meyers. Rowman & Littlefield, 1987.

Becker-Schmidt, Regina. "Frauen und Deklassierung. Geschlecht und Klasse." In *Klasse und Geschlecht*. Edited by Ursula Beer. AJZ-Verlag, 1987.

Brecht, Bertolt. "Fragen eines lesenden Arbeiters." In *Gedichte 2, Gesammelte Werke 9*. Suhrkamp, 1967.

Brecht, Bertolt. *Poems Part Two: 1920–1938*. Edited by John Willet and Ralph Manhem. Methuen, 1976.

Brecht, Bertolt. "Gedichte aus dem Messingkauf." In *Gedichte 2, Werke 12*. Edited by Werner Hecht, Jan Knopf, Werner Mittenzwei and Klaus-Detlef Müller. Aufbau Verlag/Suhrkamp Verlag, 1988.

Brecht, Bertolt. "On Everyday Theatre." In *Poems: 1913–1956*. Edited by John Willet and Ralph Manheim. Methuen, 1976.

Gilligan, Carol. *Die andere Stimme. Lebenskonflikte und Moral der Frau*. Piper, 1984.

Gilligan, Carol. *In a Different Voice. Psychological Theory and Women's Development*. Harvard University Press, 1982.

Gramsci, Antonio. "Philosophie der Praxis." In *Gefängnishefte*. Edited by Klaus Bochmann and Wolfgang Fritz Haug, vol. 6, Heft 10. Argument, 1994.

Gramsci, Antonio. *Selections from the Prison Notebooks*. International Publishers, 1971.

Habermas, Jürgen. *Theorie des kommunikativen Handelns*, Bd. 2. Suhrkamp, 1981.

Habermas, Jürgen. *The Theory of Communicative Action, Vol. II*. Translated by Thomas McCarthy. Beacon Press, 1987.

Harding, Sandra. *Feministische Wissenschaftstheorie. Zum Verhältnis von Wissenschaft und sozialem Geschlecht*. Argument Verlag, 1990.

Haug, Frigga. *Erinnerungsarbeit*. Argument, 1990.

Haug, Frigga. *Female Sexualization: A Collective Work of Memory*. Verso, 1987.

Haug, Frigga. "Alltagsforschung als zivilgesellschaftliches Projekt." *Das Argument*, no. 206 (1994): 639–658.

Holzkamp, Klaus. *Grundlegung der Psychologie*. Campus, 1983.

Kierkegaard, Søren. *The Concept of Anxiety: A Simple Psychologically Orienting Deliberation on the Dogmatic Issue of Hereditary Sin*. Translated by Reidar Thomte in collaboration with Albert B. Anderson. Princeton University Press, 1980.

Klenner, P. Christina. "Doppelt belastet oder einfach ausgebeutet? Zur Aneignung weiblicher Reproduktionsarbeit in DDR-Familien." *Das Argument* 184, no. 6 (1990): 865–874.

Kuczynski, Jürgen. *Geschichte des Alltags des deutschen Volkes.* Pahl-Rugenstein, 1981.
Leontjew, Alexei N. *Probleme der Entwicklung des Psychischen.* Athenäum Fischer Taschenbuch Verlag, 1973.
Leontiev, Aleksei N. *Problems of the Development of the Mind.* Progress Publishers, 1981.
Lefebvre, Henri. *Kritik des Alltagslebens, Band I–III.* Athenäum Verlag, 1977.
Lefebvre, Henri. *Critique of Everyday Life.* Verso Books, 2014.
Luxemburg, Rosa. *Gesammelte Werke, Band 4: August 1914 bis Januar 1919.* Dietz, 2003.
Marx, Karl. "Die deutsche Ideologie." In *Marx Engels Werke Band 3.* Dietz, 1969.
Marx, Karl. "The German Ideology." In *Marx and Engels Collected Works, Volume 5: Marx and Engels 1845–47.* International Publishers, 1976.
Mies, Maria. "Methodische Postulate zur Frauenforschung." In *Beiträge zur feministischen Theorie und Praxis, Heft 1: Erste Orientierungen.* Verlag Frauenoffensive, 1978.
Nunner-Winkler, Gertrud, ed. *Weibliche Moral. Die Kontroverse um eine geschlechtsspezifische Ethik.* Suhrkamp, 1991.
Ostner, Ilona. "Die Beschränktheit der Totalen. Anmerkungen einer empirischen Soziologin." *Ethik und Sozialwissenschaften* 4, no. 2 (1993): 252–254.
Schütz, Alfred, and Thomas Luckmann. *Strukturen der Lebenswelt.* Suhrkamp, 1979.
Schütz, Alfred, and Thomas Luckmann. *The Structures of the Life-World.* Translated by Richard M. Zaner and H. Tristram Engelhardt Jr. Northwestern University Press, 1973.
Smith, Dorothy E. *The Everyday World as Problematic.* Northeastern University Press, 1987.
Watson, Peggy. "Osteuropa: Die lautlose Revolution der Geschlechterverhältnisse." *Das Argument* 202, no. 6 (1993): 859–874.

Chapter 3

The Relation between Experience and Theory in Feminist Research[1]

Frigga Haug

The preoccupation with experience leads me to transition quickly from one discipline to another. What seems most important to feminist research is the connection between method, theory, and politics, all of which are linked to one another. In keeping with the ambivalence of my subject, *experience*, I would like to outline some considerations for our approach to experience in four sections.

Building on experience:

1 the problem of ideology
2 against "male abstraction"
3 politics and restructuring
4 responsibility

What Is Experience?—The Lived Through? The Sensuously Perceived? The Known?

We usually use the word *experience* to refer to what has been personally experienced—in contrast to theory, which formulates what is generally thought and has already been abstracted from individual experience. In everyday understanding, experience does not have to go hand in hand with understanding; yet it forms the basis of learning; it is authentic in a sense, seen with our own eyes, heard with our ears, tasted, touched, etc. We experience with our senses, which do not operate independently of the mind but in direct contact with it. What we have experienced, we know. In this respect, experience seems not only authentic but also particularly resistant to all sorts of whisperings from others, to deception and fraud. It is solid. The personal nature of experience, which we must undergo ourselves, is also strangely connected to our self-assessment. The less we think of ourselves, the more inferior our experience. It is **merely** personal. At this level, experience corresponds to opinion. One's own opinion is based on experience, yet opinion is a well-known site of ideological struggle. In this sense, experience seems especially vulnerable to all sorts of whisperings from others, deception, and fraud. The reason varies. The opposing statements intersect in the particularity of individuals. People, along with their experiences, are torn. That is why Brecht could say: *You cannot*

DOI: 10.4324/9781003480143-3

learn anything without experience, but you do not have to learn anything from experience. The contradiction formulated here outlines the problem that, in my opinion, arises in the question of acquiring social skills and expanding women's agency. After all, experiences are not simply truthful images and, as such, possible foundations of cognitive processes. Instead, the structures of this society can already be found in experiences—that is, if society is permeated by domination, its structures can be found in experience. Unquestioningly absorbing experiences would mean a simple doubling of what already exists and, thus, a consolidation of existing structures. Those already learned behaviors, such as adapting, adjusting, and submitting, would be confirmed once again; norms would be internalized. To put it bluntly, the simple introduction of everyday experiences obstructs the possibility of liberation and learning.[2]

Since human learning aims at mastering the conditions of life (i.e. at increasing liberation from dependence and surrendering to unknown powers), in a society permeated by structures of domination and vested interests opposed to too much mastery, it can be expected that the pursuit of learning, especially by women, will face a variety of obstacles at every level, preventing the necessary life skills from being gained. This occurs consistently at both an ideological and cultural level. The almost systematic incompetence concerning issues such as the regulation of social life creates anxiety and paralysis as soon as it affects oneself. Since it is impossible to live with long-term acute anxiety, individuals will try to achieve agency despite their incompetence. They do so through repression, denial, the elimination of contradictions, and their illusory reconstruction. In other words, in order to be able to act, different strategies are adopted to establish oneself within the limits, to adapt. This process also determines experience. Experience itself is, of course, already saturated with ideology; prejudices, interests, and repressive images that reinterpret boundaries are stored. However, this process of splitting the appropriation of the world is also itself experienced.

Building on Experiences—Against Male Abstractions

The women's movement stepped into this ambivalent field of experience and its conditioning with a clearly energetic insistence on experience as the starting point for personal development and science, as a weapon of critique and a means of self-discovery. The new women's movement drew this conclusion from the absence of women in all socially relevant areas and from the suspicion that this was hardly different in scientific theory, and that science and politics should be pursued as self-experience. "The personal is political"—this slogan called on many to discuss everyday problems in small groups, to move away from isolation and into the feeling of shared experience. It can be easily argued that simply exchanging experiences does not lead to understanding. The fact that accumulating stories of oppression and violence initially strengthens self-confidence but, in the long run, tends to discourage rather than enable intervention, and that self-consciousness groups always collapse after a relatively short time or, less dramatically, fizzle out, is itself a fairly certain experience within this approach to experiences. One might object that using experiences as a source of knowledge is always illusory and falsely assumes that individuals are even capable of "objectively" reporting about themselves. They process, even construct, what happened to them subjectively! Any objective validity must be denied to subjective experience. The reason: individuals twist and turn, reinterpret and distort, repress and forget what happens to them, and pursue a construction of their person to which they subordinate the content of the past. Hence, one cannot rely on what one says about oneself and how one deals with the world, for it is colored by subjectivity.

Let us turn the accusation of the purely subjective meaning of things into a research question. **How** do individuals actually change, distort, or twist the circumstances of their everyday lives, and why? The "why" is tied to their identity. That is, people rebuild the circumstances of their lives in such a way that they can exist within them relatively free of contradictions. If they cannot do this in practice, they do so in thought, in memory. So, what we can explore is not "how it really was," but how individuals built themselves into it, how they changed, what interpretations they made, what they derived from it, and, in short, how they built themselves into the existing structures.

If we want to know something about the appropriation of objective structures, it is necessary to interrogate subjective memories. In doing so, we do not assume that it is entirely at the discretion of the individual, as the connotation of the word "subjective" might suggest. Quite the opposite. How individuals perceive something, consider it good and right, beautiful and desirable, despicable and reprehensible, is the site of the daily class struggle for the minds and hearts of people. The processing of the individual, which we deciphered as the appropriation of the world and which we trace in the experiences of women, will move within the field of dominant cultural values and countercultural, resistant attempts to wrest meaning and enjoyment from life. There will be compromises.[3] In the empirical study of women's experiences, it is advisable to write down, as a kind of theoretical framework, the habits, customs, rules, and norms: what is expected, what is generally thought of, what exists in our minds as moral expectations and semi-theoretical attitudes, as well as the hopes attached to self-socialization in contrast to alien socialization. One will find that our actions, as far as we can remember them, are in a certain way at odds with social expectations and our own wishes; that is, the problems have been displaced. Examining the composition of compromises also means uncovering possibilities for living differently, discovering how life could be lived differently— where changes are necessary and possible.[4] I will give an example below.

Let us return once more to the phenomenon that women from the women's movement increasingly took for granted that theoretical work should begin with their own experiences and that theory should serve their practices. The demands formulated in such expectations appear unscientific and only legitimate if they are formulated by a member of the labour movement. It immediately becomes a problem for the scientist in question if he does not meet such demands; he cannot mediate. Behind this lies the certainty that the workers' experiences are somehow related to the science in question. Different with women. Their demands appear to want to drag science down into the trivialities of coffee chats, housewife gossip, and children's cries. Terms such as surplus value, class struggle, and production relations seemingly have no role in the kitchen. And Brecht's apt statement, that the meat in the soup will not be decided in the kitchen, reminds us once again that women's actions and experiences in the kitchen are irrelevant to the relevant social struggles; that the process only runs in one direction, from the social whole down to individual practices. The fact that vast areas of practice—the domestic-private—are, at best, incorporated into the theory of society with deficiencies such as "insufficient consumption," means that, conversely, science cannot feel at home in the domestic sphere. The claim that concepts from social production and class struggles should be applied to the family sphere appears to be a contamination of science, a detachment from social struggles. Yet this fear unwittingly reveals the legitimacy of women's protest: since Marxist science, with its claim to be a science of liberation, has so far had nothing to do with women's family practices, experiences, lives and activities within this vast social sphere, it remains uncomprehended, and its perspective, along with the question of women's emancipation, remains equally unclear. This can be seen in the different ideas and policies on the family held by left-wing men and socialist countries.

However, scientific theories and their concepts are derived from people's concrete practices. By working out regularities, they must abstract from concrete diversity. This is what gives them their power, while simultaneously creating the impression that all practices can be grasped using a terminology that does not actually apply to all of them. In *Capital*, for example, Marx analyzes wages as the value of the commodity labour power; he shows that this is determined by the value of the means of subsistence necessary to produce and maintain labour power. He then states: "Hence the sum of the means of subsistence necessary for the production of labour power must include the means necessary for the labourer's substitutes, i.e., his children..."[5] Women are not even mentioned in this sentence, and this omission symptomatically expresses their position in theory and practice. They belong to the logic of the reproduction of existence, functioning as instruments in the reproduction of capital and in social labour in the form of wage labour, as necessary as a roof over one's head or a bed to sleep in. The perspective of women's liberation thus must be further developed through additional theoretical effort and the use of different terminology.

Politics and Restructuring

When discussing feminism, experience, and theory, it is impossible not to consider their practical transgression into a liberation project. As Peter Weiss states, "Liberation cannot be handed to us, we have to conquer it ourselves. If we fail to conquer it ourselves, then it will have no consequences for us."[6] These brief words encompass all dimensions: the connection between experience and learning, personal development, understanding, and liberation. Let us jump into the current politics of liberation: if women occupy parliaments, party leaderships, trade union leaderships, and all other public areas of society, then it should be possible—so we hope, despite all critical insight into the many shortcomings of our gender—to pursue a different kind of politics: one closer to the needs of the people, less technocratic, heartless, wasteful, warlike. Behind such ideas is not the notion that women are "naturally" warm-hearted, soft, friendly, and peaceful people, in contrast to the other sex. Rather, our hope for the female dimension in politics stems from the analysis of the sexual division of labour. This is based on the separation of one area of activity from the profit-driven labour of society as a whole—waged or paid labour—predominantly allocated to men; from the transfer of all other activities—primarily the care and nurturing of people themselves—to women to be carried out for free, but under the protection of employed men; and the further separation of the regulation of this divided community into an area of professionalized politics for money and therefore, again, into a male domain. In this context, we think that women in official politics could contribute not only their experiences from the specific areas of their responsibility, thereby bringing politics down from the heights of paragraphs and life-denying decisions, but that their entry into this male domain would also disrupt the structure of the division of labour in such a way that the general reproduction of domination and oppression could not proceed in the same secure manner.

Hence, we must solve the paradoxical problem that women are largely excluded from the public sphere and politics, yet this cannot be a matter of simply growing into these structures, but instead of women overcoming the orders that oppress them in their pursuit of liberation. A further problem remains: women are trapped in conditions that imprison them in such a way that, from their personal experience, their liberation becomes an obstacle course for which they do not seem to have sufficient strength. That is, their experience also hinders the very movement of their liberation.

Experience and Responsibility

I will now link political hope with the previous reflections on the construction of femininity, the ideological formation of experience, and its consequences for theoretical knowledge. To make this connection more straightforward, I will illustrate it with an example from memory work on the topic of female responsibility. The area of responsibility is, in a somewhat unclear way, at the center of politics. It is common knowledge that women do not usually feel responsible for the larger area of official politics and world events, but instead for their private home, for the comfort of everyday life. In my experience, such common knowledge is often not entirely accurate upon closer examination. It is therefore important to study women's actual experiences with the issue of responsibility. With the aim of studying the obstacles posed to women's political engagement by the social expectation that responsibility be limited to private matters, we attempted to examine the topic of women and responsibility in a women's seminar in Hamburg, using our own experiences as a means of gaining insight. We wrote stories drawn from our everyday lives. Such stories are often unpredictably astonishing in their mixture of the expected, and therefore known, and the unexpected, and therefore forgotten. Under the title, "When I once felt responsible," we wanted to work out how individuals understand and construct responsibility for themselves; what meaning it has for them and what materials, raw materials, and connections contribute to this construction. Below, I present one such scene and its working-through.[7]

> *It was Wednesday or Thursday— so there were still two or three days until the Saturday morning shopping for the shared apartment—and the fridge was looking pretty empty. The cold cuts and cheese were almost gone, there was only one lonely slice of bread in the breadbasket, and there was only one can of cat food left. So that would definitely not last until the weekend. Anger rose within her as she had been shopping more often in recent weeks, while Anita and Werner did not seem to care whether there were always enough supplies. If necessary, they went to the restaurant... Martina did not have time today, but she had cleaned a lot over the weekend, as she often did, and had already promised to clean the bathroom this weekend. Her anger was not directed at them, because Martina regularly did things for the shared apartment and also remembered in good time to organize chores and make arrangements. Anita and Werner, on the other hand, always had to be reminded that there was still something to do. This was the case now too. They did not even think about planning the shopping. Werner worked a lot, was not home from 7 a.m. until 8 p.m., and usually had to work on Saturday mornings as well. What annoyed her was that he did not at least do something now and then - that he had less time, she realised. She was particularly angry with Anita, who said she and Martina were so dogged about everything. She had plenty of time since she stopped working.*
>
> *Her ideal was that everyone would do something regularly, that they might not be able to do all the housework, but that arrangements could be made. If the person who could not go shopping, for example, cooked a meal now and then, did something nice, such as getting cake on Sunday, or stepped in when they had absolutely no time - that would be nice. Then she could feel really comfortable and relaxed at home, would not have to think about everything constantly and could sometimes enjoy that others were taking care of her. Especially when she had a lot to do for her seminars and working groups, she would be happy if her household worries were taken care of.*
>
> *It annoyed her that she had to deal with the household's hassle and dysfunctionality instead of being able to devote her energy to her other activities. In the beginning, she had enjoyed the fact that everyone took part in the shared apartment, that a meal was ready when she got home, and that she could enjoy the care of others. This was in stark contrast to when she still lived with her boyfriend. She goes shopping.*

We turned our amazement at the banality of the story into a study of its construction. Our first question was: What does the author actually present to us as responsible actions or feelings? After some hesitation, our answer was that she went shopping for the shared apartment. The story hardly needed to be written for this conclusion; we all knew that shopping for a shared apartment was a common way to take responsibility. Yet, the author writes extensively, with a great deal of commitment and attention to detail. Behind the first answer lies a second: *I* had to feel responsible because the others did not. And so, the story revolves around the irresponsibility of the residents, which renders the shared apartment uninhabitable. Responsibility appears as an annoying compensation for the mistakes of others. In stark contrast to the lofty sentiments that the term "responsibility" usually evokes in Sunday sermons, the author teaches us that responsibility is thought of and felt in conjunction with resentment (*always me*, because the others are too lazy) and duties, agreements, organization, planning, arrangement, and above all, work. In response to our question about the context of responsibility, we encounter strict commanders (duty, organization, etc.) that ensure we must feel responsible. My sense of responsibility arises when there is a gap in the organization, so it is a kind of emergency aid. If everyone "does something regularly," no one has to feel responsible. As a first conclusion, we can say that **individual responsibility always arises when general regulations fail. And: individual responsibility is unthinkable without the simultaneous lack of responsibility from others.** The author offers two further connections: work and pleasure. Strangely enough, work is not on the side of responsibility but rather opposed to it. Those who work a lot do not have to bear as much responsibility; "because I work a lot, it is unfair to burden me with too much responsibility," she assures us repeatedly; or those who do not work should bear responsibility. There is, therefore, an emotionally agreed-upon division of labour. This is not simply the division of housework and wage labour. Rather, behind the familiar idea that housework should fall to those who do less work outside the home, the following suggestion emerges: working outside the home requires an organizational solution for matters of enjoyment, well-being, and relaxation. Where this does not happen, these areas fall into the realm of "care" and, thus, of reluctantly accepted female responsibility. We arrive at the conclusion that: **female responsibility is therefore a mistake, a social deficiency, a sign of disorder on a societal scale. What remains unregulated here are the questions of physical well-being. The disorder is exhausting.**

We finally sought to find out what answer the author actually provides to the question of the reproduction of female responsibility, which she so clearly describes as a mistake? We found three answers: **necessity** (there is no longer enough food); **anger** (there is always talk of how angry she is with the others); and finally, **anger about the anger itself**. She demonstrates very clearly that petty calculations, anger, and a lack of care destroy coexistence; yes, that the very feeling of anger is an annoying one. We concluded **that the acceptance of oneself and one's feelings, the desire for enjoyable companionship, and necessity are three forces that lead women to assume responsibility as a reluctant act.** This result points to a contradiction in the construction of femininity and female responsibility. We formulate it provisionally as follows: **the acceptance of oneself and one's feelings depends on actions one judges to be wrong.** From this story, we have gained three important insights: **first, that the reproduction of responsibility occurs through the contradictions within the person; second, that responsibility is articulated negatively; and finally, that there is an awareness that women's responsibility points to social disorder.**

I am stuck at this point. As a relaxation exercise, and because it is always beneficial to use the available productive forces, I returned to Freud. Every time I do, I am again surprised at how little interest he showed in the mental health issues that concern me. Responsibility is almost entirely absent for him. In a few places, he mentions responsibility. It is in relation to dreams. The question that preoccupies him is: Are we actually responsible for our immoral dreams? By immoral, he means those sexual fantasies that disregard the incest taboo and—in keeping with heterosexual classification—do not exclude father and brother in the case of girls, and mother and sister in the case of boys. This question stirred up emotions. Freud discusses the strong opinions that want to absolve us of all guilt and those that hold us responsible. Wisely and Solomonically, he agrees with Plato: it is better to commit outrages deeds in a dream than while awake. The hungry resentment that grips me after such a revelation is not solely due to this obsession with sexuality. I impatiently find that the tool already provided for understanding is not being used appropriately. The correct observation of a contradiction between the different dimensions of our being, which also manifests between the self-imposed demands of morality and our own actions, is missed in favor of interpreting a struggle between drive and morality. What falls by the wayside is not, as I initially assumed, the possibility of seeing morality itself as ideological and domineering but rather the struggle against it for motives other than those of the sexual drive or the Id. It seems to me that it is not so much the demands of cultural society that force us to compromise with pleasure and sexuality, with instinctual demands and their satisfaction. Although this idea—that our social life also demands a certain sadness from us—is captivatingly elegiac, in the case of female responsibility, it does not seem to me nearly resistant enough. Instead, it seems to me that the context of domination, in which responsibility plays a role, places demanding morality into a different kind of tension than just the opposition to the pressing drives. In the end, both fall by the wayside: the pleasure of instinctual life and the possibility of fulfilling moral commandments. Let us leave the sphere of Freudian sexuality and turn to female responsibility in our society. Although women are also responsible for their sexual lifestyles, what is essential to them is responsibility for the immediate well-being of their husbands and children within the immediate circle. Our subject shimmers with meaning. Seeking support from other disciplines is stimulating, albeit unsettling. According to the philosopher Hans Jonas, the principle of responsibility requires us to limit our actions to the foreseeability of their consequences. The choice of words is ambivalent, especially for women. At first glance, it seems obvious, yet ultimately too narrow. It is this limitation to the foreseeable that makes responsibility an unbearable torture for women. After all, all the dimensions in which they bear responsibility are private tasks; however, the private arrangement conceals, albeit increasingly inadequately, the fact that the means to carry them out are not in women's hands. How they furnish their household, feed and clothe their families, what education they receive, and what opportunities they have in society depend primarily on their income. But that is not all: news about the poisoning of food and air, and, not least the danger of nuclear war, make it clear that women are expected to assume a responsibility for which they are in no way equipped. The virtues required of them are those of the social community and its regulation. Wherever they try to comply with them, that is, take responsibility, they are bound to fail or deceive themselves. They become guilty. Their personal courage consists in enduring this guilt for as long as possible; the way out is to become ill. Thus, in a world that does not function, the task of preparing a tidy home against the disorder of society is experienced as an individual problem. Contrary to Freud's assumptions, attempting to intervene here would not only cause chaos and imbalance but would also be a prerequisite for liberated agency.

It seems to me that this expansion of female responsibility is the only chance to simultaneously escape individual failure and feelings of guilt and to intervene to bring about social change. Thus, fundamentally, we are not dealing with two responsibilities neatly separated by area; the task is no longer to reject the "responsibility" assigned to us by going on strike (as was proposed in the women's movement), but rather to take it up, push it beyond the surveyed area, formulate it as a claim to social power, and fight for it collectively. And of course, to generalize it to all members of society. In this respect, women today occupy a key position.

Do such considerations actually have anything to do with female identity, with experience, and with theory, or with what is expressed in this way? Women, without moving, sit at this intersection of the incompatibility of this society and individual life. They would rather allow themselves to be torn apart than relinquish or extend this unreasonable responsibility. They still experience being torn apart as a personal guilt. They take it upon themselves. The humanity that comes into their actions masks inhumanity on a larger scale. In this way, women contribute to the reproduction of their own necessity as these particular women, thus allowing themselves to be torn apart at these very seams. In addition to the legend of female masochism, which is anchored in the assumed nature of women thanks to the structure of society, a general hypocrisy also arises. On the one hand, women are seen as the good, the humane, the warm, and the sensual, for which it is worth living; on the other hand, they can be held responsible whenever something goes wrong. Examples abound: the neglect of children, school performance, drug use, cleanliness, nutrition, health, but also morality in general immorality—it is always women who have failed in something: as mothers, in the family, in raising children, as lovers, etc. Their masochism would then consist, among other things, in their attempt to live it, and the tale that transforms such attempts into a female characteristic would have the function of reassuring us that such social disorder appears solvable within the female character.

One means by which this course is set is love, along with the fact that a large proportion of women in our exchange society cannot reproduce themselves in the common currency. Where everything is exchanged for money, they earn nothing or less than they need to live. This makes their situation unpredictable and boundless, like love itself. They always give too little, and they feel that they are neither loved enough nor love enough to accomplish these Herculean feats of social order, as expressed in the maintenance of that illusory community known as the family. This, of course, is also experienced as a character weakness and guilt. Women are willing to compensate for a lack of love by redoubling their efforts.

Do such provisions actually apply primarily to women, and not also to men on the other side of that social work architecture that we call the separation between public and private? I do not mean to suggest that the male side of this context in any way represents a perspective for us, any more than the female side does. However, it is essential to include the context of domination in which the genders stand in relation to each other in the analysis, rather than (as seems to be part of the consensus, for example, after Rita Süßmuth's reform attempts[8]) viewing both genders as equally partial and as role clichés. The rewards that the social structure has in store for its male inhabitants also make it clear that they can at least pretend to have influence over the conditions of their actions. The social hierarchy sets requirements for masculinity that seem achievable and redeemable. The peace that women make with the unfulfillable demands to individually produce happiness, life, and the culture of life is this combination of guilt and masochism to the point of self-destruction.

The question of female masochism led us beyond the problem of responsibility to the question of social demands on women. As I have tried to show, consenting to being torn apart by impossible tasks leads to an attitude that we could decipher as masochistic. The attempt to assert such an attitude as inherent to femininity shifts the crucible to the level between the individual and society per se, as I showed with Freud, rather than focusing on specific social formations. I would now like to go a step further and take a final look at the benefits that this arrangement of femininity and masculinity has for the reproduction of our society. It is not just the case, as has been said louder and louder since the beginning of the new women's movement—that is, for 20 years now—that the work carried out quietly and individually by women is part of the foundation of this society and, as such, should be recognized, taken seriously, and valued. Furthermore, the general lack of responsibility for individuals in this society is lived as a mutual inadequacy of the genders. The area of life for which women are directly responsible becomes marginal from the standpoint of social production and administration— the male domain. At the same time, the activity in the area promoted by society becomes alienated, so that hopes for life are directed toward precisely that marginalized area. In this way, women are burdened with the unreasonable task of representing hope for a better life even while in a state of oppression. Certain aspects would need to be shaken up here, and a new order established.

Concluding Comments

Whenever I try to confront problems of theoretical knowledge, particularly the absence of femininity in male theories, I find myself entering the realm of social relations of domination. This path leads through the search for female experiences and their conditioning within our society. Women's experiences are essential in order to make theoretical statements of a general nature. Otherwise, science remains partial and confined to the realm of the pre-human. At the same time, however, experiences as the site where oppression is inscribed, normalized, and naturalized. We need an approach to deal with experiences that simultaneously absorbs them and takes them beyond themselves, deciphers the traces of oppression, and creates tools for liberation. Sooner or later, the entire society, and the position of women in it, comes into focus, transforming my epistemological problem into a political problem. Nevertheless, the following also seems to me imperative for feminist science and research: that it does not pursue knowledge for its own sake and its implied lack of impact but rather commits itself to attempts at liberation in every case.

Notes

1 Editors' Note: This text was published as "Das Verhältnis von Erfahrung und Theorie in feministischer Forschung," *Videnskabshistorie og-teori. Kvindeforskningsseminar* (Kopenhagen, 1989).
2 Frigga Haug, "Erfahrungen in die Krise führen oder: Wozu brauchen die Lernenden die Lehrer?" *Die Wertfrage in der Erziehung. Argument-Sonderband,* no. 58, ed. Georg Auernheimer, Irmgard Fleischhut and Norbert Frank (Argument, 1981), 67–77.
3 See Paul Willis, *Spaß am Widerstand. Gegenkultur in der Arbeiterschule*, trans. Nils Thomas Lindquist (Syndikat, 1979); Paul Willis, *Learning to Labour. How Working Class Kids Get Working Class Jobs* (Saxon House, 1977) and *Theorien über Ideologie. Argument-Sonderband,* no. 40, ed. Projekt Ideologie-Theorie (Argument, 1979).
4 For an explication of memory work in this context see Frigga Haug, *Sexualisierung der Körper. Frauenformen, Argument-Sonderband,* no. 90 (Argument, 1988).
5 Karl Marx, *Das Kapital, Marx Engels Werke Band* 23 (Dietz, 1962), 186; Karl Marx, *Capital Volume 1, Marx and Engels Collected Works: Volume 35* (International Publishers, 1976), 182.
6 See Peter Weiss, *Die Ästhetik des Widerstands* (Suhrkamp, 1975), 226; Peter Weiss, *The Aesthetics of Resistance,* trans. Joachim Neugroschel (Duke University Press, 2005), 199. Translator's Note: Peter Weiss was a Swedish/German novelist and artist. He is particularly known for his plays *Marat/Sade* (1964) and *The Investigation* (1965) and his novel *The Aesthetics of Resistance* (1975).
7 The scenario and its elaboration originate from my contribution: Frigga Haug, "Verantwortung als Masochismus," *Küche und Staat. Politik der Frauen*, ed. Frigga Haug and Kornelia Hauser (Argument, 1988), 96–106.
8 Translator's Note: Rita Süßmuth was a German politician of the Christian Democratic Union who during the early and late 1980s advocated for increased medical education and public health preventative measures.

References

Haug, Frigga. "Erfahrungen in die Krise führen oder: Wozu brauchen die Lernenden die Lehrer?" In *Die Wertfrage in der Erziehung. Argument-Sonderband*, no. 58. Edited by Georg Auernheimer, Irmgard Fleischhut and Norbert Frank. Argument, 1981.

Haug, Frigga. "Verantwortung als Masochismus." In *Küche und Staat. Politik der Frauen.* Edited by Frigga Haug and Kornelia Hauser. Argument, 1988.

Haug, Frigga. *Sexualisierung der Körper. Frauenformen, Argument-Sonderband,* no. 90. Argument, 1988.

Haug, Frigga. "Das Verhältnis von Erfahrung und Theorie in feministischer Forschung." In *Videnskabshistorie og -teori. Kvindeforskningsseminar*. Kopenhagen, 1989.

Marx, Karl. *Das Kapital. Marx Engels Werke 23*. Dietz, 1962.

Marx, Karl. "Capital Volume 1." In *Marx and Engels Collected Works, Volume 35*. International Publishers, 1976.

Projekt Ideologie-Theorie, ed. *Theorien über Ideologie. Argument-Sonderband,* no. 40. Argument, 1979.

Weiss, Peter. *Die Ästhetik des Widerstands*. Suhrkamp, 1975.

Weiss, Peter. *The Aesthetics of Resistance*. Translated by Joachim Neugroschel. Duke University Press, 2005.

Willis, Paul. *Learning to Labour. How Working Class Kids Get Working Class Jobs*. Saxon House, 1977.

Willis, Paul. *Spaß am Widerstand. Gegenkultur in der Arbeiterschule*. Translated by Nils Thomas Lindquist. Syndikat, 1979.

Chapter 4

Feminist Literature and Working with Female Experiences[1]

Frigga Haug

J. V. Uthmann writes that: "For several years now, black and feminist do-gooders have been trying to influence curricula outside of their ghetto. Their favorite target is the lists of books that many American universities require their first- and second-semester students to know."[2] While the author names "scandalous" examples, such as the inclusion of Sappho, Jane Austen, and Virginia Woolf, what makes the author shudder is the improvement of the world through literature, which gives us hope. My interest in new feminist literature lies in the questions: How is knowledge made possible as a prerequisite for the ability to act, and why is it precisely feminist literature today that takes on such a task in an exemplary manner? My thoughts focus on novels by Marge Piercy,[3] as well as Barbara Wilson,[4] and Sarah Schulman[5] from the 1980s who provide exemplary analyses of Piercy's novels.

Experience and Theory: The Political Project as a Problem of Knowledge and Communication

Theoretical discoveries are appropriate in the search for knowledge. Abstracting from colorful diversity, the *concept* conveys an understanding of the matter, provides information about the essentials, provides orientation, and allows many things to be ignored and some things to be set aside. Experience, interest, and partiality enter the process of *abstraction*. Feminist critiques of conventional terminology refer primarily to the neglect of female experiences, the resulting false universality of theory and categories, and the androcentrism of Western theory for centuries.

The long-standing problem following such literary criticism is the need to make female experiences speak, find concepts, and rebuild and renew theoretical ideas. Among other things, there lies the problem of establishing a connection between levels of experience and theory. For over a decade, we have tried to close the gap between female experience and theoretical understanding through memory work in various women's projects. The work is laborious and progresses very slowly.

By contrast, recent feminist literature offers the feeling of flying. Entire continents of female experiences open up. To gain knowledge, and for pleasure, I deal with such literature and ask how female experiences are processed, made to speak,

DOI: 10.4324/9781003480143-4

and ask what new theoretical insights can be gained from narrative. The additional fascination is that such insights and findings are much easier to convey at the level of literature than they once were or are at the level of theory.

Literature and Experience—*The Family*

In what follows, I proceed in such a way that I first make sure of those theoretical connections that, in my opinion, are discussed in the novel. Regardless of whether the authors construct their novels so that they transmit theoretical knowledge into experiences, I present the individual experiences in literature as transmitting theoretical ideas. Moreover, I examine what other insights and shifts in women's expression of their problems are made possible by working through the literature. The two topics experienced in the novels, family and abortion, are two topics in the women's movement that are as old as they are now somewhat arduous, but theoretically well thought through.

In her novel *Fly Away Home,* Marge Piercy writes about the complex process of gaining individuality as a woman. The knowledge of the women's movement is that the family form is fundamentally a prison for women. Theoretically, we could formulate that "women have to overthrow the bourgeois nuclear family in order to assert their personality."[6] However, theoretical insight into the restrictive form does not simply connect to liberating, form-breaking practice. Even where analytical sentences happily riff against personal experience, individual women are not necessarily able to connect their wishes with their thinking. Commands of liberation become unconvincing. Our theoretical assumptions relate to the construction of women as specific social and private subjects, the context of separation between public and private, the family's form of reproduction and the division of labour secured by it, and vaguely to a higher-level social structure.

Let us consider how Piercy writes about this connection: First, we meet a good-looking, happy, successful woman, Daria, middle-aged from middle-class America. She has just left her television program, in which, as usual, she skillfully presents her cooking recipes (how do I, as a working woman, prepare tasty and aesthetically successful meals for my family or my guests in just 20 minutes?) and is on a flight home to her family (husband and two almost-grown daughters). She keeps telling herself how happy she is and what a wonderful family she has, in contrast to her mother, who wasted herself on her family and allowed herself to be dominated and cheated by her husband. She was always unhappy, saving her most beautiful things for a possible other life, saving and waiting till she died. Daria herself married up. For her, there has been an unstoppable upward trend, for ever larger items and homes.

Her social life (represented by sophisticated guests at the dinner exquisitely prepared by Daria) is also satisfying. She holds no resentment that she must prepare all this food; on the contrary, she loves it; it gives her meaning. We are introduced to her family happiness over many pages. Good moods and cheerful care are presented to us until this idyll's infinite nothingness, boredom, desolation, and mendacity overwhelm us as painful reading. Then, like a bolt from the blue, the husband's decision arrives: he gives the family a lot of expensive Christmas presents (his wife gets two housecoats) as well as an application for separation—the pace of the novel changes. The wife's initial despair turns into a woman's self-doubt: What advantage does the other woman have over me? What does she have that I do not have?

Daria's feverish zeal is doubly directed. The search for the other woman, which takes place as a secret pursuit on the street and in cafés and whose discovery does not yield anything special, becomes a search for the man's actions, all the stranger the closer she gets to him. She must realize that she was never interested in her husband—as he correctly accused her—and certainly not in what he—a successful lawyer—did outside their shared home. While looking to spend money on his lover, she finds outrageous account transactions, most of which are scheduled under her maiden name and which she cannot explain. She transforms her original jealousy into an eager search for his actions in the business and political world. The woman steps out of the private gender relationship. She begins to understand gender relations as relations of production on a large scale, as a system that permeates the entirety of society.

Once the husband returns, he slides with great ease into the bedroom and bed they once shared, and just as quickly, she trusts his desire for a particularly elaborate dessert, which she spends a lot of time preparing. However, this turns out to be stupidly wasted due to the subsequent impossibility of shared enjoyment. Piercy works with the ambiguity of words. In others whom the man also defrauded, tenants whom he used every means possible to throw out, she finds allies with whose help she uncovers the worst real estate speculations and even collateral murders. Her good upbringing allows her to invite the tenants demonstrating against her husband's company into their house, where she can simultaneously prevent neighbors from discovering transgressions and thus prevent slander. The people of color, the unemployed, the poorer people, and those with a lot of children look so inappropriate in her well-ordered, thickly carpeted living room, that she herself appears out of place.

In her search for the truth, she becomes increasingly unfamiliar with her husband's business, which he started after unsuccessfully running for political office. She recognizes herself as someone who, with her hunger for the sheltered security and harmony of her home, helped produce that terrible outside world full of calculation and meanness. As the novel continues, she changes everything: her relationship with herself and others and the world, the shape of her life (more than 30 people come and go every day in her new apartment, which is much smaller than her house was), the relationship with her daughters, with her new boyfriend, and the weighting of her actions (she takes her job seriously and, unlike before, she also counts what it brings in because she depends on it); yes, even her well-mannered, temperate self transforms into a more ordinary, violent, and passionate person. She learns to use violence herself where it is necessary.

Literature and Theory

If we view literature not according to aesthetic or literary criteria but as material from which social scientific knowledge can be gained, our theoretical presuppositions about the field in which Piercy writes undergo a series of expansions, deepenings, and shifts.

First, it is believed that women's feelings for or against family are contradictory and that clear decisions and actions are impossible. Piercy writes about feelings differently. The main character, Daria, lives her individual sensations one after the other. At first, there is nothing but approval, comfort, understanding, and pride—contradictory feelings are displaced into the historically earlier figure of the mother. The fact that the daughter is happy in the same way in which the mother only felt unhappiness, preemptively undermines the possible attitude of the reader to understand happiness and unhappiness as something for which people are solely responsible, and it would therefore be important to create one's own happy, and completely different, family against the experience of the unhappy parental family. Happiness is as deceitful as the husband is a deceiver. However, Piercy does not encourage us to recognize and denounce feelings of happiness, jealousy, and betrayal as false; on the contrary, she shows that they can be kept quiet in the form of the family if the form itself holds and that only when an inevitable break occurs do they turn into false hopes against the individual. In a different arrangement that breaks down the family's anchors and possessions feelings would take on a different strength and meaning. No element or dimension is dismissed as incorrect, but they all change their importance for the main character and her life. This is the second lesson.

From the wife's point of view, as long as she is okay, her husband appears to be good, caring, and okay. Nevertheless, he can also insist at any moment that she must leave the order. As soon as he leaves her and breaks up the family unit—and immediately wants to sell the house as it is too big—her actions and attitudes, which were previously considered normal, become nonsensical, unnecessary, and wrong. On "shopping day," she does not know how much or why she should buy; she learns to live with a feeling of constant pain. Piercy transforms the familiar and thus shows how lessons can be learned. In the scene in which the tenants, threatened by her husband, stage a small demonstration in front of their house, the concept and feeling of neighborhood changes. The five people first introduce themselves as the *Save Our Neighborhood* group. "'What neighborhood? I don't understand.' One thing she was sure of was that they were not her neighbors."[7] Even in this slight hint, the term "neighbors" shows itself as a class term, and Daria knows that she is on the opposite side of those tenants who are not her neighbors. Piercy reinforces this certainty through careful, distancing descriptions of each individual from Daria's point of view and through subsequent clarification through her attack on her neighborhood. The "fat woman" says: "'We're bringing your shame home to you. You ruin our neighborhood, so we're going to cause a little trouble for you in yours.' She raised her sign and waved it. 'Come on, guys, let's make some noise.'"[8]

Home and neighborhood are not simply class concepts; their very occupation is antagonistic. Belonging determines what is appropriate for you. So, Daria immediately knows what she has to do. This knowledge, Piercy shows, is one she owes to her husband. Moreover, although he is withdrawing from her life, Daria seems particularly called upon to produce this ideal world of home and neighborhood.

> She did not want them parading in front of the house. Ross would be absolutely furious. Everybody on the street had doubtless seen them already and registered the information on the instantaneous gossip radar of the neighborhood.... It was her duty to defuse this scene... She must get supper started and she must deal quickly with them. Ross would be pleased by her quiet and efficient handling of a potentially nasty situation. She would disarm them by showing she had nothing whatsoever to hide. She would do the last thing they expected and thus lighten the confrontation and incidentally get them out of view of her neighbors. "Look, I insist there's been a mistake, but why argue out here? Come inside and let's sit down and talk."[9]

Daria employs learned phrases of politeness and decency. Within her inner dialogue, she assures herself not of her feelings but of her necessary actions based on the anticipated feelings of her husband. The aim is not to make him angry or, conversely, to make him happy. His supper must be made. Wherever her desire is mentioned, it is already found beyond her domestic neighborhood, which is now described as gossipy and controlling. Daria does what she was trained to do: turn demonstrators into guests and invite them in. In this short scene, Piercy shows that the "weapons" this woman, married, living in a good home, has, and that she still wants to use for her husband and for his protection, are reversed in the event of a crisis. Bringing non-neighbors into one's own home to hide them from other neighbors is the beginning of her transformation as one of the others. Whenever she develops feelings, she starts to question herself because immediately after she lets the strangers into the familiar, and when it becomes clear that Ross was by no means pleased by this, her act functions as further alienation and reasoning for him to spend the night away from home. She needs more information, which she can only find with the demonstrators. So, she opens her eyes to see that the longed-for normality of career, growing wealth, and power is a fraud on other people's lives, including her own. Her participation only in Ross' home life allows him to create waste in other lives, which is built into the foundation of his advancement. By being blind to the world insofar as it was not her home, she contributed to conditions in which uninhabitability, the lack of the right to a home and life, is part of the calculation of doing business for many. By renouncing herself, renunciation becomes an attitude that Ross, the husband, can impose on anyone and everyone without him noticing. She must come out of her innocence, in which she is guilty of not being a living person. It was only during the court hearing, when her feelings were no longer dominated by desperation but by indignation, that she learned that he devalued her work as a television cook just as much as she did, a circumstance that led her prudently to fit such work into his daily schedule; she cooked in advance and froze meals in small portions when she had to leave him "uncared for," while he, on the other hand, considered her earnings as insignificant toward the payment of daily expenses. So, at the time of the divorce, his own income, untainted by everyday life, also appeared to him as property to which he alone was entitled to and for which he had been saving alone, the basis for his power.

She belatedly realizes that he could always control what she earned and spent but that she never knew what he did, neither financially nor in any other ways. The banal accusation from everyday married life that one is not "interested" in the other is not confirmed as quarrelsome or unnecessary by Piercy. Instead, she shows that the accusation is justified and that such disinterest contains the possibility of everyday villainy. Here, too, insight is gained by shifting the order in which accusations and feelings are entertained. In the context of the ongoing active reproduction of oppression, we do not learn that women have false feelings or that they participate in the history of domination, but rather that through the integration of life's hopes and feelings into forms of the private family those indispensable desires for happiness, the longing for life, become dull precursors to unhappiness and renunciation of life. This not only affects individual women but also serves as a prerequisite for exploitation and injustice to flourish in general.

The method with which Piercy allows her characters to gain knowledge is, in a sense, an "embarrassment." Old feelings, reprimands, behaviors, and actions embarrass themselves in new arrangements. Daria—as in the scene quoted above—increasingly feels that she no longer knows what is "right" or, that when she acts "right," something wrong comes out of it. She becomes unbelievable in every way, even though her credibility as a wife was never up for discussion because it had no value. Only in the community of deceived tenants can words and feelings, attitudes and actions, be developed and owned. The husband must leave the house so that she can try to develop her standards, not simply reflect his anticipated expectations. In this way, we learn that our esteem and the disdain of others are connected, that the inability to respect oneself does not make one rebellious against the disregard of others. However, the inability to develop and self-confidently assert one's individuality is not impacted as long as the diverse family demands offset it. In this way, Piercy seems to mean that the gender relations protect and blind self-knowledge and, simultaneously, the knowledge of gender relations in society. Talk of love that makes you blind comes to life in such disturbing ways.

For a while, there was a discussion, particularly in the socialist women's movement, about the class or stratum to which married women belonged: that of their husbands or, because they do not have their own wealth at all, the next lowest group, or even always to that of the exploited? Although such questions were asked for political and strategic reasons, they were academic and inconsequential. However, Piercy shows, both in the novel outlined above and in other novels, that such questions about social belonging still arise in practical life. Daria, the main character in *Fly Away Home*, acquired the appropriate habitus for her marriage and the associated status that socially climbs from level to level. Appearance, temperament, education, manner of speaking, wishes, and feelings all fit together in the family like a glove.

Since almost none of these belong to her despite her social and professional activity, all dimensions stand around her like foreign bodies after her husband decides to divorce, as in the problem of the demonstrators brought into the house. Her habitus has become dysfunctional, just as she is "property" without an owner. So, she joins forces with others who are also dispossessed. The apparent male recourse to her as a possible abandoned property is initially made impossible because she moves in with a Puerto Rican woman with a child who has become homeless due to the machinations of Daria's husband. By repeatedly changing the position of "property" and its respective meaning, Piercy shows that a woman only becomes her own when she tries to gain access to property in this world (as far as they need it—for living, for example) with other propertyless people. In other relations, in which being used is a general regulator, possession as a means of power and domination becomes property in an emphatic sense. In this respect, Piercy does not make it so easy for us to take sides against property or for the dispossessed. Instead, she suggests disputing ownership in its current form. Strategically, it seems to suggest that alliances for women cannot be sought in the dominant culture through its representatives, but with all those who have somehow left the dominant culture or are not even allowed there.[10]

The diverse additional and shifting theoretical dimensions on our topic of women's oppression and family form do not come across as lessons themselves but as a narrative about a particular woman's life. This makes it lively and challenging. However, does this not simultaneously show a certain randomness and limitation, and is, therefore, still a long way from actual knowledge? Or is this not, once again, an example of the problem of how theoretical insight can be gained from individual experience? Piercy does not give us an answer to this. After all, she writes literature and not a treatise on the subject. However, we can find a possible answer from the arrangement of the literary material. The novel is written to suggest a relationship with the main character, Daria, as a woman. At the same time, this cannot happen as a simple identification. Daria continually finds herself in new constellations where her old ideas, wishes, and desires undergo radical transformations into new forms. At the same time, this makes identificatory engagement distant. As atypical as Daria's real life seems, compared with the lives of other women, it is also typical in its various dimensions of emotion and thought.

Such a scenario entails that readers can assume different subject positions. What connects us as women with the main character is the commonality of women's oppression and, therefore, the necessary and easy willingness to seek solutions. We can describe the tension that comes into the novel in this way as the fascination of solidarity. By allowing her main character, Daria, to deal with her life experimentally, Piercy allows readers to constantly compare and productively discuss their phases of life. Equality and inequality mean that the readers gain a similar distance from themselves and their experiences, as does the main character in the development process in the novel. Individuality gains a reflexive attitude. This is how women who are seized can become women who seize something.

As social scientists, we are left with the methodological question of how theoretical knowledge can be obtained from experience. Theoretical work with experiences is indeed needed to show something generalizable in experience. This complex and sometimes tedious work seems to be resolved differently in women writers. They write their own experiences so that what is worth showing emerges clearly, regardless of whether the entire narrative is fiction or directly autobiographical. In this respect, fiction is a material that almost imposes itself on theoretical work. The new feminist literature with urgent problems and questions from the women's movement is a stroke of luck, especially for feminism—that through which centuries of women's experiences must restrospectively be recovered and reworked.

Literature and Experience—Body Appropriation and Abortion

> You shall not create an ideal for yourself, neither of an angel in heaven, nor of a hero in a poem or novel, nor of one you dream up and imagine; rather you shall love a man as he is. For Nature, your mistress, is a stern divinity who haunts the girls' infatuation in women until the third and fourth age of feelings.[11]

As antiquated as many may find Schleiermacher's words, they remain highly relevant to the question of female nature and feelings. Let us here sketch one of Piercy's early novels, *Braided Lives*. Again, the theme is the development of female identity. Piercy writes: "The core of falsity in the search for love: a woman gives herself to a man as if that got rid of the problem of making an identity, with a most personal god to reward, pardon or damn."[12] For me, this is a story that tracks the possible and impossible appropriation of one's own (female) body and, in this way, is a book about abortion.

Although we are transported to the problems of adolescent girls in the 1950s, and while today's generation is, therefore, likely to have greater ease and confidence in dealing with their bodies, the problem has become more topical due to the recent discussion about § 218.[13] The questions of abortion have been stuck in the polemic of government policy for years: whether and when fetuses are/become living people, whether murdering or protecting life should have top priority, whether the "mother's" decision against the "child" should even be allowed to take place; and conversely, like an echo, the political answer comes from feminism that women's stomachs are their property and they, therefore, have the right to abortion.

Piercy begins, so to speak, by beginning with the opposite question: The problem is that adolescent women first have to appropriate their bodies in order to be able to live in them. The novel describes the apprenticeship of Jill, a daughter from a humble background who goes to college on a scholarship to escape the confines of her home and become a poet. In this space, she can breathe, learn, think, and write. She shares a room with her beloved cousin and learns from her experience with the opposite sex. They come to the conclusion that Jill will probably not be normal without some appropriate sexual experience. Such a proposition seems all the more likely since she enjoyed physically sensual games with other girls from an early age, including her cousin. She did not understand this as sexuality. The hardships of going to the cinema for the first time with other students who do not interest her begin, and finally, the intervention of her cousin introduces her to a poet. In between, there are efforts to make the body attractive without any money. Bras with cups that enlarge the breasts are stolen. The summer of rapprochement and the impossibility of finding a space in which the sexual experiment can be carried out stretches on endlessly. Finally, upon the arrival of the holidays, she borrows a car, which requires mutual introductions to each other's parents. After the doubts about whether she is deformed, because it does not work at first, to the conviction that premarital sexuality is frowned upon because it would make obvious how boring and painful it is, to regular "love" in a forest hideaway, which goes hand in hand with a consuming desire for love to the point of self-abandonment, the first year of study passes.

Piercy writes of these apprenticeship years as a constant concern with the problems of the body and the consequences of sexual love. She relates this to the status of studying, the organization of space and meetings, the perception of others, self-presentation, and the terrible monthly questions about whether one is pregnant and the almost insoluble problems of an actual pregnancy. The dominance of the body makes the question of how a love relationship between people forms fade into the background. The question becomes utterly impossible due to the exaggerated moral ideas of the parent's generation, which associate the need for marriage with the loss of virginity. Even though Jill does not want to get married, she knows that her boyfriend's similar rejection proves he does not love her.

At the center of the novel is an abortion. Here, Piercy presents this issue of public parliamentary debates and simultaneous private silence as a female tragedy.[14] It begins with an act of control. Jill is home for the holidays. She wakes up, and her mother is leaning over her dresser with the calendar in her hand, "Jill, are you with child?"[15] Unconvincing attempts at reassurance: only "thirty-two days…I am late because of the turmoil."[16] The mother only needs a few words because, as a woman, she speaks from her own experience. Piercy lets her speak of her inclusion in the female tradition as a point of pride and, simultaneously, as a knowing judgment: "You're regular, like all the rest of my family."[17] Jill retreats into a placeless resistance: "If you try to make me marry him, I leave this house."[18] At the same time, the threat is no threat, and yet behind the language, there is, so to speak, the announcement of getting completely lost. "I want an abortion."[19] The mother collects the opposing reasons from morality and law. She mixes it with class experience and with submission to patriarchal violence. The doctors "are dirty men, Jill. They charge a fortune and they blackmail you…. It is against the law. You can go to jail. Your father would kill me!…They butcher you so you can't have babies after."[20]

Against such dominance stands maternal authority and women's experiences for centuries: "I will tell you what to do." The mother's teaching speaks of survival in submission and its secret: the space for self-determination that remains in surrender is violence against oneself. Consequently, she begins her instruction with a reminder of the daughter's weakness, which she must now overcome. "You've always been a weakling and a coward. Sickly since you were seven. You'll have to do this for yourself. You'll do what I say or I'll wash my hands of you."[21] This threat draws the daughter into the chain of women's violence to which she must submit if she wants to escape other violence that comes from men and the state. The mother threatens to use male paternal power against male doctors' power, whose money motives she knows well from women's experience.

If the daughter gives her body to these specialists, she will betray the father, who will give nature its due. "I'll tell your father and he'll make you have it."[22] The mother knows the matter is hopeless: the alliance against women consists of money, law, specialists, paternal power, and female nature. The strength of women necessary for survival is the fight against their own nature, compared to all other forces which seem almost harmless. Piercy seals the entry into this women's fight with short staccato-like sentences that sound like an introduction to an ancient test of life: "Don't think it's easy. It's hard, hard," says the mother. "You'll see that I'm strong enough," the daughter replies and puts herself under the mother's authority by repeating her words: "Tell me what to do."[23]

Piercy does not describe in detail what advice the mother gave; however, she presents Jill's struggles with and her body like those in heroic tales of young men who grow up fighting dragons, liberating themselves in the process as well as others—primarily virgins. Yet Jill's fight does not take place with something outside, but rather inside her own body, in which fate is about to take place, which no willpower can overcome precisely because she is no longer a virgin. She can kill herself rather than have her body cease to be a home for something else. Accordingly, Piercy chooses the inner monologue form and sets individual words in vain opposites. Jill waits until the tub has filled with hot water:

> I sit in the toilet seat staring at my belly smooth and flat from harsh laxatives. Under the cushion of fat lurks the womb, spongy fist that will not open while in it cells divide and divide. The steam swirling hot from the tub smothers me as this body goes its animal way.[24]

Jill must realize that the animality that clutches her is, in fact, herself as a woman.

Within her gendering, all previous hopes of being human become ridiculous mirages.

> I seldom felt feminine: I felt neutered. An angel of words. I could imagine myself a Hamlet, a Trotsky, a Donne. I thought I was projects, accomplishments, tastes: I am only an envelope of guts. This is what it is to be female, to be trapped. This sac of busy cells has its own private rhythms of creation and decay, its viruses

> and cancers, its twenty-eight-day reminders of birth and death. My body can be taken over and used against my will as if I were a hall to be rented out. Hot baths with Epsom salt, hot baths with penny-royal; I am parboiled and still pregnant.[25]

Shakespeare had Hamlet go to a churchyard and talk about the transience of life and the takeover of the dead by worms. How can the hero overcome death?

Piercy shows in the banality of the bathroom that for women, death is in their lives, that they are vessels of ceaseless growth and, therefore, constant death. This is how women enter history as species-beings. Jill continues to talk to herself:

> Like my mother to cuddle a dark-haired girl-child and suckle it on my frustration and beat it for my hunger and bind it for my loneliness. To sacrifice myself for a girl-child whom I will try to teach to sacrifice herself, a chain of female suffering.[26]

In the increasingly hot air, her thoughts become confused "sick dreams." Jill feels that the power that has come against her is also love. Not only the love for her boyfriend, a seduction to which she succumbed, but the love for the life that arises within her, against her, and which is, at the same time, her death.

Piercy also organizes the drama by trivializing this field's usual and "normal" questions. In the middle of this catastrophe of realizing that Jill is a woman as a body and with her entire life, the parents suddenly appear, as does the boyfriend, to discuss questions about a possible marriage and, in particular, whether Jill's background is middle-class enough for Mike's middle-class parents. The mother defiantly points out that she owns a small house and a well-preserved car that is only two years old. Thus, she moves away from Jill's world and becomes herself a path that cannot be trod.

Jill must finish her fight. The mother calls on her again: "You aren't trying hard enough."[27] She shows courage to fight and jumps from higher and higher furniture until it becomes clear that she has to end it differently. By this point, she had lost 20 pounds, but the being within her remains triumphant. She tries to steal away its apartment and stabs herself in the chest with a knife. The injury is only minor, and she realizes that this is just a game.

> Now I will go to work attacking my body in earnest... Thursday night. I am half dead and nausea is a constant state, my heart is beating erratically, and yet I am still pregnant. Upstairs in the hot and airless attic, I prepare to follow Mother's last instructions. Through the floorboards the hoofbeats and gunshots of a Western arise. 'Don't cry out', my mother warned me. 'Keep your mouth shut'. Squatting in the ruins of my old sanctuary, by force I open my womb.[28]

Piercy ties the ends of her story back together. The small space on the floor that was a retreat, a possession, a place full of secrets and possibilities, the treasure of Jill's childhood, had become too narrow for her plans. She needs more air to breathe, space to think, people with whom to discuss, and to "change the world." The way out is also how she realizes what it means to be a woman and experiences herself as a woman. The metaphors get in the way of each other. In a room that is too small, she knows there is another small room within her which takes up her space. She must enter this in order to be able to step out of the chain of women's fates. The means is violence. There is no alternative. Jill almost dies in this act. So, what she did is not a generally recommended solution, but it is nevertheless necessary.

Piercy shows other women's fates as impossible paths: there is their first beloved friend from her school days who becomes a stranger to her when she gets married at 16 and has a child. Now, she is serving a life sentence in prison because she shot the man who had thrown the child down the stairs. A college colleague has child after child to hold onto the man who ultimately leaves her anyway. There is another student who is expelled from college because she has sexual relationships with women. And finally, there is the love of her life, Donna, her cousin, who wants to combine marriage and work, but must have an abortion and dies because of it. This final shock puts an end to all dreams. At a time-lapse pace, Piercy brings the currently possible solutions to an end: Jill must give up her wedding despite it already having been announced. Disturbed, she disappears for a time from every conscious and rational life; then, she organizes an emergency service for women who must have abortions because otherwise they cannot survive as human beings. One tool she uses to achieve this is to blackmail doctors who have performed illegal abortions.

The book does not offer definitive solutions but instead draws us into the various dimensions that need to be discussed about abortion as questions of women's ability to appropriate the female body. There is no easy way to grow into the body and become social with it. Even with the first sensual impulses related to another body, questions of normality are at stake. The cultural pressure, especially from people of the same age, in heterosexual relationships quickly comes up against questions of legality. The parents additionally monitor both normality and legality. The breach of parental trust is not just a moral question. It leads to new, far more dramatic danger zones. Contraceptives are not safe; if abortion is illegal, it costs so much that for a long time, one's entire life must be devoted to organizing money, in addition to the physical problem and the carefully guarded secret. The reality of pregnancies not only ends the departure into a possible life of one's own, but it also teaches that in our patriarchal culture, a woman's body becomes a trap for her. However, she can no more survive as a conscious, sensuous being without the attachment of the body than she can with it.

What remains? Finally, the long-term struggles in the women's movement have at least made abortion options easier to the point that the means Jill resorted to are no longer commonplace. Despite all the bigoted discussions about reinstating the criminalization of any abortion, the needs and practices of the generation of women described above belong to our history, no longer to the present. However, this novel about female apprenticeships reads like a condensation of the same questions about the female body and its appropriation by us and others. There is still a struggle for solutions through which to gain the different dimensions of life: for love without giving up oneself, for the body and its sensuality without losing it or turning it into a mere carrier of further life against one's own will, without oneself having a life.

Once again, I ask myself what insights this literary approach to female experiences has given me. I could list several dimensions whose connections had previously escaped me. However, the most important thing is the position that knowledge itself has. These novels consist not so much in the sum of new knowledge, not in results, new connections, and discoveries, but rather in how readers are involved. It becomes clear that knowledge cannot be anything external to us and something gained in itself; it is the process in which we are actively involved. In dealing with the last novel, for example, I encounter Piercy as meaning that there are many open questions to the problem of the female body and its "humanity" but no real solutions yet. These cannot be sought in exchange with the male sex because, concerning these female bodies, it acts as a kind of executor of natural history or morality and law, for example, if the person involved is ready for marriage and fatherhood.

Although the body belongs to each individual, it is a problem for the entire female gender. It is, therefore, a necessary historical practice that women's experiences are passed on and acted on their basis. However, these experiences are themselves embedded in the history of female oppression and natural history. Women are only slowly emerging from violent relationships. Again, women get together and organize emergency services, using existing knowledge and combining it with what they consider necessary. The legalization of abortion is still a long way from solving a sensuous and livable relationship between women and their bodies. Important advice by women remains necessary. The female future must still be won.

The insight I was looking for is that novels encourage readers to acquire knowledge about themselves and their relationship to their bodies, gender relations, and the world and to begin this process as a significant discussion. They are an attempt to raise awareness of the history of female humans.

Maybe one can agree with Sarah Schulman that marginalized people know how they live and how people of dominant culture live. However, people from a dominant culture only know how they live. The people in power have the least information. While Schulman writes about subcultures, outcasts, the self-excluded, lesbians, and gays, Marge Piercy teaches us that in a society where women do not belong to the dominant culture, precisely because it is male, forming cultural alliances with all those who also do not belong to the dominant culture is imperative. From this point, it would be possible to gain some of the necessary knowledge about women and their socialization from feminist literature and comprehensive knowledge about human socialization in general. One will be able to read that the topics addressed by feminist literature cannot simply be understood and dismissed as women's issues, and yet women are needed to address these topics of life and death, of AIDS and politics, of war and fascism, of ordinary crimes as well as of extraordinary ones, appropriately that is, in terms of their actual scope and meaning for people.

Notes

1 Editor's Note: This article was first published in *Das Argument* in 1992. See Frigga Haug, "Feministische Literatur als Arbeit mit weiblichen Erfahrungen," *Das Argument*, no. 193 (1992): 334–350.
2 Jörg Von Uthmann, *Frankfurter Allgemeine Zeitung*, February 19, 1992.
3 Translator's Note: Piercy is an American novelist and poet whose work is rooted in her Jewish heritage, Marxist social and political activism, and feminist ideals. She tends to write in first person narrative form. Piercy remains a staunch anti-war activist, environmentalist and feminist.
4 Translator's Note: Wilson is American writer, editor, publisher, and translator. She cofounded the independent feminist publishing house, Seal Press in 1976.
5 Translator's Note: Schulman is an American novelist, playwright, nonfiction writer, screenwriter, gay activist, and historian.
6 Frigga Haug and Kornelia Hauser, "Zeit für mich – über das Privatisieren," *Subjekt Frau. Kritische Psychologie der Frauen* (Argument-Verlag, 1988), 14–64, 59.
7 Marge Piercy, *Fly Away Home* (Summit Books, 1984), 109.
8 Piercy, *Fly Away Home*, 109.
9 Piercy, *Fly Away Home,* 109–110.
10 In other novels, she deals with the various groups of the left from the 1960s to the 1980s, with urban Indians, conscientious objectors, terrorists, and socialist students. Her central characters often emerge from a diverse mix of peoples, with their beauty reflecting the proportions of those who are particularly discriminated against ethnic groups—such as Jewish-Asian or Indian-Irish, Black-Chinese, and so on.
11 Friedrich Daniel Schleiermacher, "Idee zu einem Katechismus der Vernunft für edle Frauen," *Schleiermacher-Auswahl*, ed. Heinz Bolli (Siebenstern, 1968), 274.
12 Marge Piercy, *Braided Lives* (Fawcett Books, 1982), 249.
13 Editor's Note: "§ 218" refers to Section 218 of the German Criminal Code (StGB). Since its introduction in the 19th century, it has regulated the criminalization of abortion. The so-called abortion debate in Germany has revolved precisely around this section: whether, under what conditions, and within which time limits an abortion is exempt from punishment or remains a criminal offense. In short, "§ 218" is the legal core of German abortion regulation and thus the central point of reference in political and feminist debates about it.
14 Piercy, *Braided Lives*.
15 Piercy, *Braided Lives*, 208.
16 Piercy, *Braided Lives*, 208.
17 Piercy, *Braided Lives*, 208.
18 Piercy, *Braided Lives*, 209.
19 Piercy, *Braided Lives*, 209.
20 Piercy, *Braided Lives*, 209.
21 Piercy, *Braided Lives*, 209–210.
22 Piercy, *Braided Lives*, 210.
23 Piercy, *Braided Lives*, 210.
24 Piercy, *Braided Lives*, 211.
25 Piercy, *Braided Lives*, 211.
26 Piercy, *Braided Lives*, 211–212.
27 Piercy, *Braided Lives*, 214.
28 Piercy, *Braided Lives*, 218.

References

Haug, Frigga. "Feministische Literatur als Arbeit mit weiblichen Erfahrungen." *Das Argument*, no. 193 (1992): 334–350.

Haug, Frigga, and Kornelia Hauser. "Zeit für mich – über das Privatisieren." In *Subjekt Frau. Kritische Psychologie der Frauen*. Edited by Frigga Haug and Kornelia Hauser. Argument-Verlag, 1988.

Piercy, Marge. *Braided Lives*. Fawcett Crest, 1982.

Piercy, Marge. *Fly Away Home*. Summit Books, 1984.

Schleiermacher, Friedrich Daniel. "Idee zu einem Katechismus der Vernunft für edle Frauen." In *Schleiermacher-Auswahl*. Edited by Heinz Bolli. Siebenstern, 1968.

Chapter 5

Women Live Resistantly[1]

Frigga Haug

I

> When Riva was still quite small, she had already a formidable will. Even as a baby she would swell with anger, she would scream herself sick or hold her breath till I was frantic with fear. At two, she would say *No* at top volume. I can see her yet standing in the middle of the courtyard saying that one word until the walls rang and then going stone mute and refusing to speak at all.[2]

This foreshadows how Riva's path into the world will be one of multifaceted resistance. This story is told by Marge Piercy. Riva rebels against being a daughter with all the loving and hating submission that goes with it against a certain learning, against the home, against the expectations of becoming, as a woman, a wife and then a mother; "she created no channels through which my wishes and anxieties could reach her," says the mother, and sometimes I wonder "if I did not commit some early error that made love unimportant to her no matter how freely offered."[3] Overall, Riva fights against the forms of being a female member in a society in which property, which also includes women, is theft and exploitation, and life is a random moment in the organization of profit. She becomes an information pirate—one of the most wanted criminals by transnational corporations. She spies and reveals, for example, the composition of important medications to the general public, thereby making it almost impossible to generate extra profit from them in the future.

II

This outlines a broad framework of tension in which the life of woman is constantly being reshaped in many different ways. The various movements condense into catastrophes, happiness and misfortune, struggles and resignation. Alexandra Kollontai (1872–1952), an activist in the Russian Revolution of 1917–18, goes down in history as someone who fought for women's economic independence. This sounds necessary, although somewhat lifeless and insignificant. Let us read what is essential to her. Following in the footsteps of the "new woman" in the literary

DOI: 10.4324/9781003480143-5

works from the revolutionary period, she writes: "The new woman not only rejects the outer fetters, she protests 'against love's prison itself'," "she is fearful of the fetters that love, with the stunted psychology peculiar to our time, lays upon lovers."[4] And later: she is "[f]ree as the wind, lonely as the grass on the steppes. She is dear to nobody. No one will protect her."[5] In her, "too, a limit is set to her adaptation to the beloved. Her atavistic inclination to self-denial, to self-alienation and dissolution in love, collides with her already developed, distinct human personality."[6]

Love again appears as a focal point of revolt and adaptation, as longing, as danger. Love is evidently something to be desired and guarded against like fire: a temptation to self-extinction, an obstacle to the possibility of becoming a free person, and yet a promise of happiness. Does love possess us before we become aware of the danger? Or are we thrown into it as if into a prison from which we cannot free ourselves without outside help—or, because it also means being completely taken care of, do not want to? Do we seek love only to find our unhappiness in the process?

III

Such contradictions are invitations to embark on a journey of processing. Everyone is probably familiar with the diverse self-help literature and perhaps also theories that accompany women on their path to love. Let us also try to remember how we actually learned to navigate around this fire that threatens to consume us. But no matter how understandable the messages about love may seem, the question of memory immediately strays into strange territory. My first response is negative: pain. My earliest memory is of not having been loved, or at least not enough. Jealousy of my brother or sister for my mother's love, fear at school that my friend might turn to someone else—but worse still, looming over everything, was the early fear of failing precisely at this self-evident and natural aspect of loving; namely, of not being able to truly love at all. Love enters my life as a lack, but even more so as my own inadequacy. I do not really want to be so close to the friend with whom I share everything, but I suffer from the fact that others in my class in school stick together, hardly appear individually, and constantly exchange secrets and gifts. Yet, in my search to do the same, I could not find anyone who inspired in me the urge to close off from everyone else. In short, none of them appealed to me enough. Thus, my desire was directed toward every new girl who joined the class—which happened every three or four months—and I became enthusiastic and tried to establish the closeness that corresponded to the desire. After a few days, I was always thrown back onto myself. The feeling from the first hour did not last. The love object failed. An inability that constantly came pounding back to me. In the end, did I really lack the innate ability for love that everyone else had, the capacity that makes a relationship exclusive and permanent?—In my memory, I was in a state of constant infatuation, from which nothing followed but a hunger for something I could not achieve.

This got worse when the opposite sex came into play. Some of my classmates—I went to an all-girls high school—began to form tight-knit groups in the schoolyard, where heated discussions would ensue, and as soon as I joined, a significant silence would follow. Somehow, I knew they were talking about boys, and I could not contribute to such topics. Then came the time for dance lessons, which I remember purely as martyrdom. There was an expectation from which I saw no escape: each girl had to win over one of the boys from the neighboring high school so that he would become her partner for the prom and graduation dance. It began with girls and boys standing in separate rows, facing each other across the dance floor, scrutinizing one another—until the boys were asked to choose a partner. Just like in real life, a back-and-forth race immediately began for the most beautiful girls and those who could bring the most prestige; in short, even this spontaneous choice was made strictly according to economic class, interrupted only by outstanding beauty and grace, which, however, also required the appropriate clothing. I was chosen late, by someone who obviously could not find anyone better, which was no surprise since, for me, he also had nothing desirable about him. However, I was glad that someone had come along at all, and I accepted generously and with embarrassment, as if I had actually had a choice. Even today, looking back more than 50 years later, I still feel the shame of not having performed well in my first gender competition, a setback that befell me without any involvement on my part. As a kind of resistance, I initially decided to find the opposite sex boring and objected to any nightly strolls on the "Sigh Island," so-called because sighs of love were supposedly heard there all the time. From then on, I belonged even less to the inner circle of the class, which I rationalized to myself as meaning that I did not want to belong anyway, although I constantly hoped to be chosen by them. At the same time, I rationalized my exclusion to myself with external circumstances: I was a student driver, so I had to take the train home before the time of sighs. Of course, there were boys on the train with whom I tried to adorn myself. I began making up stories about relationships I did not have and was thus gradually able to improve my reputation in the class.

After graduating from high school, I was supposed to attend business school to become a secretary, as my mother, a single parent of four children, did not think she would be able to manage having all of us go through college. "You absolutely have to go to university," my classmates urged me. "Where else are you going to find the right husband?" The pretext somehow flattered me and, if I agreed, I could smuggle myself into normality and hide the fact that I did not really know what or where I wanted to go.

At first glance, the university is a marketplace for coupling. During the summer semester, which was my first, the potential brides and grooms constantly showed up wearing less and less clothes and speaking in increasingly clever-sounding ways, twisting and turning until it was time to try things out. "Dates," as they are now commonly called, could be made for various reasons. You do not have to wait for someone to choose you, as in dance class; as a woman, you could take the initiative yourself. But what does all of this mean for love? I think I was now constantly infatuated again: with the possibility of being free to do whatever I wanted without knowing what that was; with the reality of spending nights talking and skinny-dipping; with the city, which concealed unheard-of, threatening, and therefore all the more fascinating secrets. One of my first dates with an older student (he was at least four semesters ahead of me, and I only remember that he studied law), who took me to a trans bar. There, I fell in love with everyone except my companion, whom I mainly feared because I assumed that I would have to do his bidding in return for the night stroll he financed—although the scope of possible actions was completely obscure to me here as well, my imagination not venturing beyond what I pictured to be hideous kisses. I was enthralled by the variety of seminars and lectures and intoxicated by the many students whom my mother had advised me to treat as my brothers. However, I felt the same way with them as I once had with my girl friends. Seeing them, I plunged into an exuberance of emotions that lasted two or three days, dominated my thoughts, and left me in a constant state of intoxication, so much so that I had difficulty concentrating in lectures. Within a short period, however, whenever the novelty wore off, any emotional commitment deflated just like a balloon that had let out its air: in short, ordinary young men soon left me unmoved. This went on for a while. I collected friends like stamps, without much to show for it. Not even an album. And once again, doubts began to grow inside me: was I ultimately sick? Incapable of love?

Because, as I had known for a long time, love was, after all, a wildfire, so burning that everything and everyone else disappears like an afterthought.

In short, I first encountered the love Kollontai described as a prison, as a lack, then as a longing that remained unfulfilled, while the promises around me grew, giving rise to a sense of guilt and the need to conceal the shortcomings felt as failure. At some point, I experienced the increasing pressure to place life on a regular track. Overly high hopes had to be set aside; normality is the order of the day, even in dreams. Marriage is public proof that one is capable of love.

IV

The imaginary: We sense the ground on which the desire for love in its specific form, namely, focused on the search for a man and the formation of a family, is prepared with our participation. The pioneers include romance novels, which today are also adapted into films for television. The prince that is hoped for has evolved little from the fairy tale of *Sleeping Beauty*. You wait. He should come like a revelation. You will recognize him at first glance, or at the first kiss. However, another tension enters the world of imagination, which we call the imaginary. The male world not only offers hopes of awakening, but above all, poses a threat that only one's own man can protect against. This begins early on, when one must be warned about the "strange uncle" long before sexuality is discussed. Fascination and fright entwine around real figures, and this becomes even stronger the longer the game of hide-and-seek lasts. Popular romance novels, which at least until recently were devoured by young women in droves, play this same tune. In her 1984 study, Janice

Radway from the U.S. found that women borrowed up to four romance novels a week from public libraries[7]; the pattern, which appears to be addictive, as Tania Modleski explains, is essentially always the same. The "heroine" occupies a subordinate position, preferably as a maid—potentially available day and night, or in danger of being overpowered by him, the master of the house, who is the older, wealthier, or in any case, superior man, usually from another class. He pursues her inexperienced innocence and wants to subjugate her according to his experience. Therefore, she is constantly at risk of losing her innocence, even as she is on guard to preserve it. Pursuit and flight determine the narrative until the middle. At that point, the man is worn down. He falls in love with his potential victim and proposes to her. She immediately agrees, because now submission and rape are transformed into love and marriage. Her steadfastness has transformed his animal nature into a higher one. Happy ending.[8] Modlewski does not assume that a mass of women is so stupid as to simply like this repetitive pattern and throw themselves into it. Rather, she shows that readers of such novels derive their pleasure and, accordingly, the formation of their own desires, from the fact that, unlike the heroine in the book, they know from the outset—precisely because they already know the pattern—that the man's strange, brutal and cynical persecutory behavior is by no means merely puzzling and reprehensible, but rather a sign of love to come. The satisfaction derived from such novels, Modlewski thinks, comes from thoughts of revenge.

> The man should realise that he needs the female heroine and suffer for it. This realisation usually only comes after some dramatic event—the heroine has run away, wants to kill herself or almost died. These revenge fantasies have two sides: they are, at the same time, an expression of the real suffering of women under conditions of life in a patriarchal society and a protest against it.[9]

Equipped with such dreams, there remains little substance from which to win life for oneself. So, after just these few moves, we realize that it is less love itself that ensures the long-term subjugation of women, as Kollontai assumes, than the desire for love. Fueled by the embers of unimaginable expectations and growing drives, it offers little solid ground for resistance. Rather, it is a gateway for the promises whispered from all sides. In this way, the imaginary is constructed so that every insufficiency, every lack, fuels self-doubt or provokes resistance, which in turn promotes the growth of unfulfillable dreams.

"I am not talking about carnal pleasures, although there is much to be said about them, nor about infatuation, about which there is less to be said," says Bertolt Brecht.

> The world would get by with these two phenomena, but love must be considered separately, since it is a production. It changes the lover and the beloved whether for better or for worse. Even from their appearance, lovers look like producers and of a high order. They show their passion, they are uninhabitable, they are soft without being weak, always looking for friendly acts they could perform

> (not just, in their perfection, for the beloved). They shape their love and give it a legendary quality as if they were expecting a historical description. For them, the difference between no mistake and making just one mistake is enormous—a distinction the world can happily ignore. If they turn their love into something extraordinary, they have only themselves to thank, if they fail, they can just as little excuse themselves with the mistake of the beloved as can leaders of the people with the mistakes of the people. The obligations they accept are obligations to themselves; nobody could be so severe over breaching the obligations they undertake. It's the nature of love as of other great productions that the lovers take many things seriously that others treat casually, the slightest touches, the smallest shifts of emphasis. The best succeed in harmonizing completely their love with other productions; then their friendliness becomes something general, their inventiveness useful to many others, and they support everything that is productive.[10]

Let us agree with Brecht that love is not something that happens to one from the outside, like being struck by a lightning bolt, but rather an activity—comprehensive, indeed almost a perspective in a different society shaped by love. Looking back at the women in our play from the perspective of new hope, we find them first arriving in marriage, then endowed with children. Their desire for love has led them to become housewives as a first stop.

V

My own memories of this are entirely unruly and sad. As a young wife, I was, first and foremost, a student. We married not because of Brecht's grand production, but because, at that time, traveling together without being married still involved considerable difficulties, especially of a moral nature. I remember with panic how, once, a porter in a modest hotel in Italy asked us a question using the word "matrimonial," and I fled the building, convinced he was asking for our marriage certificate rather than whether we wanted a double bed or two singles. We had to travel with very little money and did not want to run into problems with our morals. And we also liked each other. So, we got married.

A student marriage places few demands on being a woman. I neglected all housewife duties and presented this as a political strategy. That worked well, until a daughter was born. Someone had to earn money; we could no longer live hand to mouth, and so the well-known division of labour, agreed upon and yet natural, began. I spent the unhappiest years of my life in a village not far from Cologne, without a degree, with a child, as a housewife, waiting alone for my husband to return home. I was used to being around many people—now there was a landlady, overly interested in snooping around, which I feared because I could always be caught in my inadequacy. Every now and then, a neighbor would stop by, cheerful and loud, asking me to clean the windows; what would the neighbors think otherwise?

This period was rich in instructive experiences for our question of female resistance. I tried out its various forms for two years. I became sick. When the man I had married came late in the evening, he would find me in my nightgown on a nearby scaffolding in the bitter cold. I did not know exactly whether I wanted to catch pneumonia, was simply looking for my husband from above, or if I initially wanted to face him but then decided that the longer the wait went on, the more I would hold out in order to get sick. I sought the withheld other, which became increasingly vague the more I missed it, by fleeing to another city. I tried to fall in love with others. I refused to do any housework. I started drinking alcohol in the morning. I thought my life was ruined. I was trapped. One Sunday, he asked me what I actually did all day. Without hesitation, I answered: I read Proust's *In Search of Lost Time*—and, as soon as I said it, I knew I had to end it all. But how?

I had no degree, no money, but a child. Because of the daughter, I was trapped, which made me love her even more desperately and think of her as the last thing that was truly mine. Returning to my mother or siblings was out of the question. So, I found salvation in the next marriage, and I handed myself over from one man to the next, taking my child with me. All the forms of resistance I had previously practised had weakened me. Above all, they had pushed my self-esteem to a point close to annihilation. Escaping into the new, old form of marriage was by no means a goal, but only the beginning of a life in which all the steps had to be relearned, all the tasks measured, and new resistances carefully acquired so they could be useful to me. The women's movement helped here.

VI

The unhappy course of many young marriages, divorce rates, and the exclusion of housewives from everything they had learned, wanted, and dreamed of is presented in diverse, stimulating, and instructive ways by many authors in world literature.

Virginia Woolf writes angrily about the emptiness and futility of women's imprisoned lives at the beginning of the last century.[11] Marge Piercy vividly discusses the futile fixation on the family, which is the case even when a woman holds a small job, because this fixation causes her to close her eyes to the world, such that she does not even notice her own husband's crimes, let alone the injustices in society in which she lives complacently. She must change if she wishes to survive. Resistance is directed against oneself, against the female form as an accessory to a man or a family.[12] In *The Longings of Women*, Piercy brings together three women whose lives are initially separate: the rejected wife of a businessman, "helping family members," who has learned nothing herself and whom he can discard once he has accumulated enough money to get a younger woman; another, the constantly cheated wife of a professor, who also teaches and who hopes that old age will calm him down enough in their marriage that he will stop taking possession of students who, in relation to her, are getting younger by the year; and finally, a student who has learned from experience that it is not her actions but only marriage that can lead her out of poverty. The three lives are brought together in such a way that, from their unfinished stories, a possible liveable life can be invented and created together. The path leads out into the world, not back into the house.

Finally, in her novel *The Summer Before the Dark*, Doris Lessing portrays a woman in her forties, Kate, who comes to realize that her family no longer needs her. The novel begins as follows:

> A woman stood on her back step, arms folded, waiting.
>
> Thinking? She would not have said so. She was trying to catch hold of something, or to lay it bare so that she could look and define; for some time now she had been "trying on" ideas like so many dresses off a rack. She was letting words and phrases as worn as nursery rhymes slide around her tongue: for towards the crucial experiences custom allots certain attitudes, and they are pretty stereotyped. *Ah yes, first love! ... Growing up is bound to be painful! ... My first child, you know ... But I was in love! ... Marriage is a compromise.... I am not as young as I once was*. Of course, the choice of one rather than another of these time-honoured phrases has seldom to do with a personal feeling, but more likely your social setting, or the people you are with on an occasion. You have to deduce a person's real feelings about a thing by a smile she does not know is on her face, by the way bitterness tightens muscles at a mouth's corner, or the way air is allowed to flow from the lungs after: *I wouldn't like to be a child again!* Such power do these phrases have, all issued for use as it might be by a particularly efficient advertising campaign, that it is probable many people go on repeating *Youth is the best time of your life or Love is a woman's whole existence* until they actually catch sight of themselves in a mirror while they are saying something of the kind, or are quick enough to catch the reaction on a friend's face.

A woman stood on her back doorstep, arms folded, waiting for a kettle to boil.[13]

The woman now really tries to remember. She continues to find worn-out phrases, little experience, where there was life, things started, abandoned, postponed—she leaves the house in search of everything: love, herself, her possible place in society, and society itself.

VII

During the era of the women's movement, in the early years of my professional life—when my daughter was already six—I puzzled over the contradiction of being a housewife. I sought to understand how women could actually manage to navigate such contradictory demands: to be human and, at the same time, to give themselves up entirely to caring for their husbands, children, and the household—and sought to identify the blockages that prevented women from standing up against them.

I knew from my own experience that this housewife's life was neither simply coercion nor just a matter of free choice. It became increasingly urgent to carefully remember women's paths, to follow their history, in order to channel possible and expected resistance into viable effectiveness.

In one of the many women's groups where I seriously examined my life and wrote and edited memories,[14] we quickly discovered that all the typical assumptions about women's persistent classification and subordination, including those we ourselves believed, were inaccurate. It was not conflict aversion, timidity, or fear that prevented us from terminating this division of labour, in which one person moves out while the other experiences the home as their main sphere of activity. Rather, it was mainly the resistance to parents and family that led to the founding of our own families, in which one would do everything differently. Resistance against the ideal of the caring mother, and against our own mothers, led to such neglect of all self-care that, ultimately, out of a pure will to survive, the only recourse left was to flee back into the role of mother. The strangest thing was that it was precisely the women among us who appeared confident and self-assured, and therefore not simply willing to submit to a man, who invested their energy into shaping his life path and did not work on their own life plans. Even here, one can still see women actively working to strengthen the structures that constrain them.

Paul Willis investigated why sons of unskilled labourers become unskilled labourers themselves. He concluded that it is the resistance to school and its semi-transparent system of regulations that ultimately condemns boys to submission. The self-destructive forms of resistance among girls showed specifically different processes of subjection.[15] In Bettina Heintz and Claudia Honegger's "Lists of Powerlessness: On the Social History of Female Forms of Resistance," for example,[16] forms of protest are not only presented as strengthening submission to the desired female mold—as when the stylization of women as weak, hysterical, prone to migraines, indisposed, etc. is met with resistance, which in turn uses illness as a means of escape, thus reinforcing the problematic image of women. Heintz and Honegger are interested in how various spontaneous forms of resistance against unhappy lives in assigned gender roles, such as those of female citizens in emerging capitalism, contributed to the consolidation of women's roles and modernization. They assume that women's lives, with the figure of the bourgeois homemaker as a perspective, even if it does not correspond to reality (i.e., even if the woman is employed), are torn apart by the following contradiction:

> The division of the world into a realm of love and the arena of competition finds its counterpart in the strict separation of the sexes, which reduces women to the home and leaves the public sphere to men. The bourgeois family, which establishes itself as a 'work-free' sphere of pure humanity, needs a cult figure who is both its producer and its symbol... The woman, once desirable and lively, is now moralised and demoralised, deformed by becoming the 'good mother,' cut to half of her person in the private interior of the nuclear family.[17]

"Female identity constitutes itself as a lack"; "only in the surrender of herself does the woman find herself."[18]

Caught in this contradiction with themselves, women set out to create the family as a counter-world to heartless economics and rationality, while simultaneously economizing it according to rational standards: the family as a business with order, hygiene, cleanliness training, and efficiency. From here, that is, from the family's inner world of morality, socio-political campaigns led by women, by "moral crusades," against the moral decay of society emanated. Resistance, therefore, is not a good thing in itself, nor its outcome always welcomed.

VIII

Psychologist Carol Gilligan wrote the bestseller *In a Different Voice*,[19] in which she essentially seeks to prove that women have a different moral code, one that values caring, from men, who carry banners of justice and principle. Ten years after the book's publication, Carol Gilligan concluded that women are fundamentally divided in this society—she calls it "dissociated." As adolescents, girls have experiences that society interprets differently from the way they make practical sense of them. During adolescence, they must decide whether they "want to know" or be "accepted" as belonging. Or, to put it another way: socially accepted ideas of a good woman, a good girl, a good mother, a good relationship, and so on, do not correspond to their own insights into social contexts. As a result, they end up in a state where they do not (want to) know what they know. Or, in other words, they must give up their personality in order to keep it. In such paradoxes, they "dissociate" themselves. Gilligan examines girls' stories for traces of real experience and concludes that women cannot integrate into this society without losing themselves. Revolt is called for.

IX

As adults usually address children, I once asked my five-year-old niece what she wanted to be when she grows up. Unlike me at that age, her dream had long been established: a veterinarian. Just two years later, she wanted to become a veterinary assistant, assistant to her husband, who would be a veterinarian. I was not only horrified but also felt superior to such premature renunciation. I had studied myself, even if I had paused when the child was born; I had written drafts for a television program for my husband, based on which he finally found a job that supported us. I had followed him, and by my late twenties, I was beginning, little by little, to take control of my life. I was already 40 the first time I refused to attend a conference as an accompanying wife. The resolve in which I persevered brought large stretches of loneliness, as Alexandra Kollontai predicted. Yet it was precisely in this solitude, in this self-chosen letting go, in this isolation, ultimately, in my own room, which I had moved into at that time, that I began to build myself into the world as my own person, with my own areas, thoughts, and plans. Once again, I needed illness, escape, and a beloved friend to see this through with me. What helped me was a university regulation that seemed to be invented against women: married couples could not be appointed to the same university. So, I built a second home in different places, travelled around the world, and came back. All of this demanded so much energy that I only began to produce the love that Brecht so insouciantly places at the beginning of life when I had been remarried for decades, when I was finally able to shape my own life. This, too, is a task that must be fulfilled every day. Thus, I finally turn Kollontai's effort to free women from the prison of love into the task of shaping love itself so that the prison that also held them captive is torn down.

Notes

1 Editor's Note: This essay was written by Frigga Haug for the women of Laichingen on the Swabian Alb on July 21 of 2004, on the occasion of the tenth anniversary of their Working Group on Feminist Theology.
2 Marge Piercy, *Er, Sie und Es* (Argument Verlag, 1993), 99; Marge Piercy, *He, She, and It* (Fawcett Books, 1993), 80.
3 Piercy, *Er, Sie und Es*, 273; Piercy, *He, She, and It*, 229.
4 Alexandra Kollontai, *Die neue Moral und die Arbeiterklasse* (Verlag Frauenpolitik, 1977), 39; Alexandra Kollontai, "The New Woman," *The Autobiography of a Sexually Emancipated Communist Woman* (Herder and Heder, 1971), 89.
5 Kollontai, *Die neue Moral und die Arbeiterklasse*, 12; Kollontai, "The New Woman," 57.
6 Kollontai, *Die neue Moral und die Arbeiterklasse*, 20; Kollontai, "The New Woman," 66–67.
7 See Janice Radway, *Reading the Romance: Women, Patriarchy and Popular Literature* (University of North Carolina Press, 1984).
8 See Tania Modleski, *Loving with a Vengeance. Mass-Produced Fantasies for Women* (Routledge, 1990).
9 Frigga Haug und Brigitte Hipfl, *Sündiger Genuss. Filmerfahrungen von Frauen* (Argument Verlag, 1995).
10 Bertolt Brecht, *Me-ti. Buch der Wendungen*, Prosa 2, Gesammelte Werke 12 (Suhrkamp, 1967), 571; Bertolt Brecht, *Me-Ti: Book of Interventions in the Flow of Things* (Methuen Drama, 2016), 160.
11 See Virginia Woolf, *Drei Guineen* (Frauenoffensive, 1978) and Virginia Woolf, *Die Jahre* (Fischer Taschenbuch, 2002); Virginia Woolf, *Three Guineas* (Random House, 1992) and Virginia Woolf, *The Years* (Hogarth Press, 1937).
12 Marge Piercy, *Fly Away Home* (New York, Summit Books, 1984).
13 Doris Lessing, *The Summer before the Dark* (Vintage Books, 1978), 1.
14 Sünne Andresen, Evelin Gottwaltz, Kornelia Hauser, Jutta Meyer-Siebert and Sabine Zürn, "Weibliche Lebensperspektiven und Männer," *Der Widerspenstigen Lähmung. Kritische Psychologie der Frauen,* Band 2, ed. Frigga Haug and Kornelia Hauser (Argument Verlag, 1986), 7–40.
15 Paul Willis, *Spaß am Widerstand. Gegenkultur in der Arbeiterschule*, trans. Nils Thomas Lindquist (Syndikat, 1979); Paul Willis, *Learning to Labour: How Working Class Kids Get Working Class Jobs* (Saxon House, 1977).
16 See Claudia Honegger and Bettina Heintz, *Listen der Ohnmacht. Zur Sozialgeschichte weiblicher Widerstandsformen* (Europäische Verlagsanstalt, 1981).
17 Honegger and Heintz, *Listen der Ohnmacht*, 31.
18 Honegger and Heintz, *Listen der Ohnmacht*, 33.
19 See Carol Gilligan, *Die andere Stimme. Lebenskonflikte und Moral der Frau* (Piper, 1984); Carol Gilligan, *In a Different Voice. Psychological Theory and Women's Development* (Harvard University Press, 1982).

References

Andresen, Sünne, Evelin Gottwaltz, Kornelia Hauser, Jutta Meyer-Siebert, and Sabine Zürn. "Weibliche Lebensperspektiven und Männer." In *Der Widerspenstigen Lähmung. Kritische Psychologie der Frauen, Band 2*. Edited by Frigga Haug and Kornelia Hauser. Argument Verlag, 1986.

Brecht, Bertolt. *Me-ti. Buch der Wendungen*. In *Prosa 2. Gesammelte Werke* 12. Suhrkamp, 1967.

Brecht, Bertolt. *Poems from the Brecht Collection: The Brass Purchase*. Translated by John Willett. Methuen, 1987.

Brecht, Bertolt. "Fragen eines lesenden Arbeiters." In *Gedichte 2*, 108–109. Suhrkamp, 1997.

Brecht, Bertolt. *Me-ti. Book of Interventions in the Flow of Things*. Bloomsbury, 2016.

Gilligan, Carol. *Die andere Stimme. Lebenskonflikte und Moral der Frau*. Piper, 1984.

Gilligan, Carol. *In a Different Voice. Psychological Theory and Women's Development*. Harvard University Press, 1982.

Haug, Frigga, and Brigitte Hipfl. *Sündiger Genuss. Filmerfahrungen von Frauen*. Argument Verlag, 1995.

Honegger, Claudia, and Bettina Heintz. *Listen der Ohnmacht. Zur Sozialgeschichte weiblicher Widerstandsformen*. Europäische Verlagsanstalt, 1981.

Kollontai, Alexandra. *Die neue Moral und die Arbeiterklasse*. Verlag Frauenpolitik, 1977.

Kollontai, Alexandra. "The New Woman." In *The Autobiography of a Sexually Emancipated Communist Woman*. Edited by Iring Fetscher and Translated by Salvator Attanasio. Herder and Herder, 1971.

Lessing, Doris. *The Summer Before the Dark*. Vintage Books, 1978.

Modleski, Tania. *Loving with a Vengeance. Mass-Produced Fantasies for Women*. Routledge, 1990.

Piercy, Marge. *Er, Sie und Es*. Argument Verlag, 1993a.

Piercy, Marge. *He, She, and It*. Fawcett Books, 1993b.

Piercy, Marge. *Fly Away Home*. Summit Books, 1984.

Radway, Janice. *Reading the Romance. Women, Patriarchy and Popular Literature*. University of North Carolina Press, 1984.

Willis, Paul. *Spaß am Widerstand. Gegenkultur in der Arbeiterschule*. Translated by Nils Thomas Lindquist. Syndikat, 1979.

Willis, Paul. *Learning to Labour. How Working Class Kids Get Working Class Jobs*. Saxon House, 1977.

Woolf, Virginia. *The Years*. Hogarth Press, 1937.

Woolf, Virginia. *Drei Guineen*. Frauenoffensive, 1978.

Woolf, Virginia. *Three Guineas*. Random House, 1992.

Woolf, Virginia. *Die Jahre*. Fischer Taschenbuch, 2002.

Chapter 6

Lesbian or Heterosexual

Heroines for Our Liberation[1]

Frigga Haug

The editorial question posed to me is: *what might be the differences between lesbian and heterosexual heroines in feminist crime novels?*[2] Although this peculiar fixation on sexual practice—especially when used to identify the category of "alternative heroines"—immediately appears strange (after all, we do not typically differentiate women categorically according to, say, their eating and drinking practices), we nonetheless understand that such a question is linked to critical hope. Whether women live in traditional gender relationships or love other women determines more than just their sexuality. Which figure, then, can be more crystallizing for women's liberation? Do we need the possible radicalism of lesbian women, or is less upheaval, as perhaps expressed in more heterosexual heroines, sufficient?

Among other things, the presentation and portrayal of positive female characters in crime novels opens up alternatives for women in the present by illuminating which paths are also possible, what women can do, what obstacles must be overcome, and possible pathways which can and cannot be taken. In these respects, heterosexual heroines are presented with specific problems and solutions that are immediately relatable for most readers. To a certain extent, such crime fiction heroines, much like their readers, live an average, everyday life, however unusual their actions may be. They often have families, or at least one or even several children. Marriage, pregnancy, and a relationship with a man are the themes interwoven with the crime story, at once determining the motives of the crime and the investigation, inspiring what is sought, missed, and punished as justice. Perhaps one could say that heterosexual heroines are more popular for a cultural-political project than lesbian heroines—they juggle problems similar to those faced by most readers: what distinguishes them from each other, and thus, establishes them as "historical personalities," as heroines, are their specific ways of dealing with their respective conflicts. To solve a crime, they must *be* something other than what they usually would be as ordinary women: more fearless, more versatile, highly qualified, and able to put their qualifications to use. Moreover, they must have developed the ability to act in all contexts despite the various barriers imposed by motherhood, marriage, and family. In short, they must be women who, despite their social positioning as women, manage to leap into alternatives, raising awareness as the criminal contexts become clearer and changes appear on the horizon. Essentially, such

DOI: 10.4324/9781003480143-6

crime characters solve the problem that people, as children of their circumstances, can scarcely be different from those circumstances, yet must be in order to traverse them.

An excellent example of this is P.M. Carlson's[3] heroine Maggie Ryan, who has accompanied us through four crime novels. Maggie is not only beautiful, athletic, musical, and very smart—she is a statistician, an amateur detective, and she is full of romance. Over the course of the series, she gradually acquires a husband and two children. The actions of this growing family play a role in the crime narrative. For example, scenes in which the baby's nappy has to be changed in the midst of hunting a criminal are impressive—actions slow down accordingly and become recognizable as possible and relevant everyday actions of women—and contrast with James Bond, who forgoes even going to the toilet for hours, even days, when hunting fever strikes.

Another typical heterosexual heroine is Claire Malloy, as portrayed by Joan Hess.[4] She is a bookseller, the mother of a 14-year-old daughter, and, of course, an amateur detective. The fact that she is a mother is not simply a biographical detail (as might be the case with being a father) but determines the entire plot. Her daughter traverses the crime scene, not only revealing the everyday female life that we would otherwise never find in a crime story but also exploring possible mother-daughter alternatives to the sometimes-fraught nature of this relationship.

Ros Howard is different again, but undeniably heterosexual, as penned by author Susan Kenney.[5] She is alternative in that she is able to occupy a place that was not usual for women within existing social patterns. She is a professor of literature and is undoubtedly qualified; she is also beautiful, young, and romantic which embroils her in significant challenges yet forces her to use her intelligence and her physical skills (she can ski, sail, and so on) to uncover the case and thus save herself. She often has difficulty coming to terms with her feelings. As she searches for the criminal, she falls in love with him, without any warning system to rationally protect her. Here, too, readers can seamlessly identify themselves with Ros' character, having themselves experienced the unreliability and separation of feelings from reason. Ros also successfully solves a challenge that all women under patriarchy face.

It becomes immediately apparent that the cultural struggle women experience must also encompass their everyday lives; that is, there is an affinity between the struggle of the fictional heroine and that of the everyday real woman. This would be tackling feminist-cultural politics through crime novels as a dimension of liberation. In this respect, we could say that our initial question about difference is answered, though in an evaluative way: heterosexual heroines are not only different from lesbian heroines, but also more impactful for women entrenched in the wider cultural-political project. Yet, why is it that readers prefer lesbian crime heroine novels over heterosexual heroine ones? But before we conclude that crime novels are more compelling the closer they are to the everyday lives of readers, let us look at "typical" lesbian heroines.

First, there are many surprises to be found when looking through many lesbian crime novels. As expected, family, marriage, the husband-wife relationship, and children tend not to play a role. However, the search for one's childhood, the question of what one has become, and the exploration of subjective barriers and possibilities are central. This applies to the tough Caitlin Reece[6] as well as to Stoner McTavish[7]; it determines the approach of the incredibly hardened private detective Michele Knight and is even built into the overall plot of Barbara Wilson.[8] Might we conclude from the figure of the lesbian heroine that detachment from everyday patriarchal struggles releases frustrated energy now redirected toward the exploration of women's own becoming and possibilities of womanhood? This seems to be a common thread throughout these novels. At the same time, one may often doubt whether the protagonist's narrative process is carried out in a sufficiently liberating manner. Nevertheless, this is always revealed as a possibility and often accompanied by alternative ways of dealing with oneself. Usually, it enables heroines to see and experience their bodies as ego, as life, and therefore also as ability. Lesbian heroines almost always master at least one type of physical combat, which they use for self-protection and in the name of the just cause.

Along with heterosexual heroines, lesbian heroines are also romantic, but sex is primarily portrayed as a fun everyday life practice, like eating and drinking. For a while, I believed that the long, inevitable sex scenes in every lesbian crime novel were intended as acts of liberation and, by being slightly pornographic, they increased marketability. After further examination, it also seems to me that they are a means of experimentally breaking the close connection between romance and sexuality, which tends to cause such disastrous blockages in ordinary women's lives.[9] The release from women's ordinary lives enables the conquest of other spaces. Barbara Wilson's heroine, Cassandra Reilly, is a globetrotter; she travels alone all over the world. However, other heroines can similarly decide at any given moment whether they want to stay or go, where to spend the night, when to eat and drink, with whom to live with, and so on; they inhabit spaces of freedom that are a mere longing for most women.

One of the cultural achievements of female writing is the gaze cast on women. Women no longer appear as exhibits, sex objects, and other objectifications. Instead, we mostly learn something human about them: what they do, where they go, what relationships they enter, what they want and can do, and so on. In some crime novels, we come to know what individual characters look like—their waist size, breast size, and so on—which are indispensable characteristics in the patriarchal crime fiction tradition. This relationship between viewer and gaze changes again in surprising ways in crime novels with lesbian heroines. After all, the heroines relate to other women as sexual beings. To make this fully clear, we need appropriate descriptions that can be immediately deciphered as sexist. For example, Michele Knight herself has "underpants with a gaping alligator mouth. You know where"[10] and describes another character, a customer, as follows: "She was blonde with a pearl necklace. Plus, a tastefully conservative grey suit. Her hair was tastefully styled, her shoes and handbag—tastefully, of course—coordinated."[11] She adds: "The same customer later stands there topless and has two well-rounded breasts, not two meters away from me. Some like breasts, some like butts, I like whatever is sticking out in my direction. And they were sticking out."[12]

At first glance, it may seem that we have sought a different perspective on women only to end up in the same place: women as commodities, clothing racks, and sex objects. Nevertheless, politics lies in exaggeration. It is precisely because all the stops are being pulled out and all *clichés* are allowed to appear that the whole scene becomes subversive. The radical "male" gaze on women, staged from the lesbian position, can be undermined and revealed as ridiculous. What occurs is the demonstration and confirmation, as well as the shattering, of *clichés* between sexual partners. It becomes clear in such scenes that they are, so to speak, the pinnacle of criminal, or at least objectifying, relationships, and by no means the perspective *per se*. In this way, "lesbian" heroines or lesbian crime novels work on other dimensions of patriarchy, certainly on biographies and on sexual relationships as relations of domination. The leap into radically different circumstances has two further advantages: it provides temporary relief from the banality of everyday life, enabling a more expansive view that offers greater capacity for action while simultaneously providing the ever-present possibility of escape. This view highlights sexual relationships, which are usefully understood as fateful, to be personal decisions, thereby suggesting greater freedom. It is obvious that we cannot uphold the hasty judgment that "heterocrimes" are more politically and culturally compelling because they relate more closely to everyday life. In such a complex and deeply entrenched structure as patriarchy, however, it is more important to constantly approach it from new points of view. Anything that deviates from the norm is subversive.

Notes

1 Editor's Note: This text was originally published in German as "Lesbe oder Hetera – Heldinnen für unsere Beifreiung," *Fama: Feministisch-theologische* no. 4, 1994.
2 For this article, I am referring to several crime novels from the *Ariadne Series*. There are also pragmatic reasons for doing so. As editor of this series, I am familiar with not only the 60 novels that have been published so far but also with the additional 60 in preparation. I chose to focus on this series, especially since Ariadne itself is comprehensively diverse, particularly given that the distinction between lesbian and straight crime stories is part of our question.
3 Translator's Note: Patricia McElroy Carlson is an American writer of mystery fiction whose mysteries include feminist themes.
4 Translator's Note: Joan Hess was an American mystery writer also writing under Joan Hadley.
5 Translator's Note: Susan McIlvaine Kenney was an award winning American short story writer and novelist.
6 Translator's Note: The Caitlin Reece book mystery series were written in the 1990s by Lauren Wright Douglas & Annabeth Albert featuring private investigator, Caitlin Reece, a witty, smart lesbian detective.

7 Stoner McTavish is a lesbian, travel agent and reluctant private investigator. The series was written by Sarah Dreher during the 1980s.
8 Barbara Wilson is the pen name of Barbara Sjoholm, an American writer, editor, publisher, and translator.
9 Surprisingly to us, this intense connection between sex and romantic love is little or not present in the crime novels from the former GDR. Still, lesbian relationships do not play a role. See the exemplary Dagmar Scharsich.
10 J.M. Redmann, *Mississippi* (Argument Verlag, 1994), 32.
11 Redmann, *Mississippi*, 8.
12 Redmann, *Mississippi*, 12.

References

Carlson, Patricia McElroy. *Audition for Murder*. Avon, 1985a.
Carlson, Patricia McElroy. *Murder Is Academic*. Avon, 1985b.
Carlson, Patricia McElroy. *Murder Is Pathological*. Avon, 1986.
Carlson, Patricia McElroy. *Murder Unrenovated*. Bantam, 1987.
Carlson, Patricia McElroy. *Vorspiel zum Mord*. Translated by Andrea C. Busch and Almuth Heuner. Argument Verlag, 1990.
Carlson, Patricia McElroy. *Sicher ist nur Mord*. Translated by Andrea C. Busch and Almuth Heuner. Argument Verlag, 1991.
Carlson, Patricia McElroy. *Versuch mit Mord*. Translated by Andrea C. Busch and Almuth Heuner. Argument Verlag, 1992.
Carlson, Patricia McElroy. *Makler und Mord*. Translated by Sigrid Sengpiel. Argument Verlag, 1994.
Douglas, Lauren Wright. *The Always Anonymous Beast*. Naiad, 1987.
Douglas, Lauren Wright. *Lauernde Bestie*. Translated by Else Laudan and Martine Osburg. Argument Verlag, 1989.
Douglas, Lauren Wright. *Ninth Life*. Naidad, 1990.
Douglas, Lauren Wright. *The Daughters of Artemis*. Naiad, 1991.
Douglas, Lauren Wright. *Sieben Leben*. Translated by Eva Stäbler and Martin Grundmann. Argument Verlag, 1993.
Douglas, Lauren Wright. *Töchter der Artemis*. Translated by Eva Stäbler. Argument Verlag, 1994.
Dreher, Sarah. *Stoner McTavish*. Translated by Martina Friedrich and Else Laudan. Argument Verlag, 1990.
Dreher, Sarah. *Stoner McTavish*. New Victoria Publishers, 1985.
Dreher, Sarah. *Something Shady*. New Victoria Publishers, 1986.
Dreher, Sarah. *Gray Magic*. New Victoria Publishers, 1987.
Dreher, Sarah. *Stoner McTavish 2 Schatten*. Translated by Else Laudan and Martin Grundmann. Argument Verlag, 1990a.
Dreher, Sarah. *Stoner McTavish 3 Grauer Zauber*. Translated by Monika Brinkmann and Else Laudan. Argument Verlag, 1990b.
Haug, Frigga. "Lesbe oder Hetera – Heldinnen für unsere Befreiung." *Fama: Feministisch-theologische Zeitschrift*, no. 4 (1994): 10–11.
Hess, Joan. *Strangled Prose*. St. Martin's Press, 1986.
Hess, Joan. *Dear Miss Demeanor*. St. Martin's Press, 1987.
Hess, Joan. *Rufmord*. Translated by Adelheid Zöfel and Gerlinde Schermer. Argument Verlag, 1992.

Hess, Joan. *Liebe Miss E. Tadt*. Translated by Adelheid Zöfel. Argument Verlag, 1994.
Kenney, Susan. *Garden of Malice*. Penguin, 1983.
Kenney, Susan. *Graves in Academe*. Viking Penguin, 1986.
Kenney, Susan. *Zuchtrosen*. Translated by Argument Verlag, 1992.
Kenney, Susan. *Tod nach Lehrplan*. Translated by Argument Verlag, 1993.
Redmann, Jean Marie. *Death by the Riverside*. Naiad, 1990.
Redmann, Jean Marie. *Mississippi*. Translated by Monika Brinkmann. Argument Verlag, 1994.
Scharsich, Dagmar. *Die gefrorene Charlotte*. Argument Verlag, 1993.
Wilson, Barbara. *Gaudí Afternoon*. Virago, 1990.
Wilson, Barbara. *Ein Nachmittag mit Gaudí*. Translated by Else Laudan, Eva Stäbler, and Martina Friedrich. Argument Verlag, 1992a.
Wilson, Barbara. *Trouble in Transylvania*. Seal Press, 1992b.
Wilson, Barbara. *Trubel in Transsylvanien*. Translated by Birgit Albrecht. Argument Verlag, 1994.

Chapter 7

Victims or Agents?[1]

Frigga Haug

The question posed in the title, "Victims or Agents" seems somewhat silly in itself. Either I choose the alternative "agent," in which case I would be as outrageous as the judges in trials who want to prove that women play an active role in rape; or I agree with the alternative "victim," a solution that can build on so much consensus that my contribution would already be over at this point. It would not be worth dwelling on the question any further. Because it is clear to everyone: women are primarily victims. There is plenty of evidence to support this: women's shelters, the countless numbers of women who have been raped and assaulted. Then, there is the fact that women are not allowed to pursue certain professions. They are kept out of public life. They are not allowed to enter the temples of power. They eke out their daily existence in subordinate and auxiliary or entry-level occupations. They are underrepresented in interest groups. They are doubly burdened by the chaos of housework and screaming children, while their husbands indulge in watching television, drinking beer, bowling, flirting with their secretaries, experiencing exciting adventures, and endlessly climbing up the ladder of success. There is no doubt that women are victims. Mostly, they are victims of their husbands, but certainly of social conditions. Their public reputation is poor. Take advertising, for example. Parts of women's bodies are used in many ways to stimulate purchasing desires; they serve to heighten emotions, for example when a girl in shorts or just a girl's bottom is exhibited sitting on a motorcycle, which together are intended to encourage the purchase of a particular brand of cigarettes; or when beer can only be sold with breasts—right through to the aesthetic design of products, such as ashtrays shaped like a woman's belly, a nutcracker replicating a woman's thighs, etc. Their reputation is equally low in the workplace. How they have to work and what people think about it are illustrated by a remark from a personnel manager who was otherwise quite amiable and humane. We asked about the requirements for computer work, and he replied: "If the potential errors are known and the testing program can run routinely, then it's just plain prison labour and can be done by women." And another: "Our women must be able to stand well, be resilient, and be under forty. They must not be too corpulent, not like Italian Mammas."

In short, women's work is generally considered synonymous with unskilled labour. This very roughly summarized evidence for the view that women are

DOI: 10.4324/9781003480143-7

victims of these conditions and victims of men can also be found in most feminist literature and characterizes their point of view. Thus far, and I can only agree: women are oppressed in our society.

What can be done about this? How can they stand up?

There are—to put it briefly—two obstacles to such standing up. First, the oppressed bear the marks of their oppression. This means, for example, if we want to extract reality from the words of the personnel manager: the women he employs probably do not have the same skills as the men working there because they cannot draw on the same work experience. So, today's women cannot do everything. Second, women have difficulties in their struggle for their own liberation because, under certain circumstances, they may not want what they want. This means that those who are on the move, those who want to liberate themselves, are not only fighting against external obstacles, but also face additional difficulties with themselves, for example those commonly known or discussed as relationship problems, which hinder the revolutionary impulse. In this context, I use the term "relationship problems" to refer to downplayed breakdowns in women who are unable to cope with private conflicts, which render their attempts at liberation impossible.[2]

The question I now ask myself is: what are these structures, these social conditions in which women are oppressed and from which they bear the marks of this oppression? I can give a very brief answer here because this connection is generally known. Women are primarily there for the family. The family is still considered the fundamental unit of society in which women are expected to ensure the protection of their offspring. I will now refer to being a woman, being a housewife and mother, reproducing men, raising children, and giving up one's life goals and every other purpose in life, in the abbreviated form, as the social function of women.

This function is commonly linked to women's nature. First of all, it can be said that this is not unjustified, since, after all, women are the ones who bear children. This quick argument is immediately followed by the doubtful question: Is women's nature so overwhelming, or, in other words, are they so unable to regulate their nature that it must become the content of their lives? The question I now pose to myself is: What is the relationship between the "domination of nature," which is so highly regarded by society and has already been pushed so far, and the nature of women? Simplified and translated back to our previous question about the natural constraint of women's social function, this also means: Do women actually have to have so many children that their entire lives are filled with and dominated by them? The question seems ridiculous, but a cursory glance at history shows that this has indeed been the case up to a time that is frighteningly close to the present. I will provide only two examples here—as sufficient material can be found in several existing research reports[3]: First, more precise knowledge about contraception has only been gained in this century. Second, the possibility of not breastfeeding children—a strenuous activity that tied mothers down for one, two, three years, or even longer—required the sterilization of food, which was only discovered at the end of the 19th century. Until then, that is, until the beginning of the 20th century, women who lived with a man might give birth to as many as 19 children, less than half of whom survived. (Incidentally, the legendary craftswomen who are often discussed in the women's movement, i.e., female butchers and other women organized in guilds, also gave birth to a very large number of children, meaning they were practically constantly pregnant). The rapid growth of society through such behavior, despite the high infant mortality rate, was, as is well known, mitigated by the fact that not all women were allowed to marry and, in such social exclusion (monasteries), not all women gave birth to children. When women have 19 children and then have to breastfeed them, leaving little time or opportunity to undertake anything else (it goes without saying that after 19 children, or even after 18 or 17, they are likely to die in childbirth), one can certainly speak of an extreme level of being at the mercy of one's nature. This kind of subjugation of women to their own nature has become unnecessary and superfluous with the development of contraception and the possibility of raising children with "foreign food." Nevertheless, women are kept in the family as if the same relation still existed. At this point, I am not trying to speak out against breastfeeding in general. However, it seems to me that knowing and examining exactly where women are hindered by their own nature in a society where a cultural form (the family) simultaneously binds women is important for any desire for liberation. One's own nature must also first be appropriated, and breastfeeding can only become a pleasure if it does not have to be done month after month, year after year.

The function of women in the family is an obstacle to their development; it excludes them from essential areas of society, makes them dependent, and is oppressive. Beaten down in this way, denied rights, and degraded to fuel consumption, women are exiled to the kitchen stove and additionally abused for public amusement. In the form of jokes, the unanimous laughter agrees: women are evil, stupid, useless, and vain. Their activities are consistently portrayed in a negative light. Entire books could be filled with jokes in which women appear only in the reflection of their husbands, such as this one: "Fred is asked, 'Are you married?' and he replies, 'No, I just look it because my car was stolen.'"

But there are not only such jokes that one dismisses, feeling mad and angry. Since women are constantly exposed to such misogynistic jokes, they usually just turn away in annoyance without giving the joke a second thought. However, in my attempt to find such jokes as evidence of women's poor public reputation, I discovered a peculiar, somewhat different additional meaning. I will now present three such jokes, which can probably be considered typical misogynistic jokes:

"The student driver says to her driving instructor, 'I always drive through red lights because green does not suit me.'"—We are supposed to laugh at the claim that women are mainly concerned with clothes and appearances. Another Jewish joke: "A husband tells his friends: 'My wife is really clean; she is the only person in New York who cleans the trash before throwing it away.'" –The joke forces us to jump back in history to understand it, because the agreement to laugh at such a brainless act by the woman has long been superseded by the practice now actually required in times of waste separation and recycling; namely, to do just that: clean the trash before disposing of it.

Or a third joke from ÖTV magazine: a picture—sunshine, meadow, water, a couple on a towel with a portable radio. The man looks worried, the woman angry. She says, "I told you right away: turn off the news on such a beautiful day, but no, you are sulking and thinking about overkill."

I think that such jokes, despite the superficial, petty agreement to make fun of women, are also critical jokes. They contain an enlightening moment. They show that the areas in which women find themselves and the activities associated with them must be destructive to women themselves. This applies both to the silly joke about the driving instructor, in which the woman chooses to drive through red lights and to the joke about overkill, which she ignores because she wants a cozy, cheerful atmosphere. And it even applies to the joke that highlights the futility of cleaning, precisely because such labour is now outdated. In other words, even at their most malicious, these jokes are enlightening; they say something about the threats that these areas, which are the "realm" of women, pose to women. Through exaggeration, they distort the conventional, thus pointing to the need to liberate women from "their realm." How would such liberation and change be possible? Does it not require—and do not these jokes also suggest this—women who have already been changed?

Let us remember that existence in marriage and family life, motherhood for women, implies extraordinary restrictions, dependence, and hindrance to development. If every woman knows this, how is it that they still desire motherhood and marriage? Another choice is possible. Women are not forced into it. To put it more strongly, I now formulate the following thesis: by wanting, or at least secretly desiring and striving for, motherhood and marriage, women voluntarily consent to their submission.

In a series of jokes, such as the ones just quoted, two things become clear: on the one hand, wasted lives, and on the other hand, that women are beginning to fight back within these areas, but that this resistance is aimed in the wrong direction. As proof, I will quote a clearly misogynistic and tasteless joke that nevertheless illustrates these two points: "Some women are like cigarettes. In the end, the poison accumulates in the mouth." Such jokes indicate that women are beginning to fight back in this shunted life, albeit in a distorted way that is not aimed at real liberation. This obviously requires an understanding of the construction of the oppression into which women voluntarily enter. How does it take hold of women?

For further analysis, I propose the following thesis: Any oppression that does not operate with external coercion must rely on the consent of those involved.

The assumption presented at the outset, that women are exclusively victims, proves hopeless if one wants to fight to change their situation and at the same time insist on their participation in liberation. It remains forever in the dark why liberation is possible and necessary, and above all, who should accomplish it, or rather—to put it more generally—how women, as victims and objects, can actually attain the status of active subjects. In other words, the view that women are exclusively victims remains silent about how they can move from being in the position of those who are acted upon to the position of being agents themselves. If women clung to the idea of being victims, stamped and sealed, they would have to remain silent, they would have to stay in place, and they would not be able to rise up from their oppressed position.

If, on the other hand, one assumes that people, and therefore also women, are creators of themselves, then it follows that individual women find the structures of oppression, the social conditions in which they grow, in which they are expected to adopt a slouched posture, already in place. But these structures only exist if they are continually produced by those who live within them. This also means that these structures can be changed by those who produce them. This, incidentally, is the only way in which change can be conceived. That is, the idea that women can change their own relations presupposes that they also partake in producing these relations; therefore—as claimed above—that oppression, if and insofar as it does not operate through external coercion, requires the consent of the oppressed. Every action, therefore, contains a degree of consent. Even self-sacrifice is an act and not fate.

If we accept the imposition of considering such consent to oppression, the question arises as to how such acts of consent come about. A tentative answer: in the process commonly referred to as socialization, what happens is not a simple stamping, the imposition of certain character traits from above, as a number of socialization theories claim, but rather the process of socialization is itself an activity in which consent must be produced at every stage. How can this happen? I will now outline some assumptions from critical psychology.[4]

We assume that the development of individuals, the growth of children into adults and every further development, is a process of constant uncertainty. One learns something, achieves a position of knowledge and agency, and is inclined to remain secure at this stage. In order to continue growing, to reach the next stage, one must abandon the old stage that has just been achieved. This is a process of uncertainty, or, in other words: a conflict. Reaching the next stage requires resolving the developmental conflict and, in turn, itself offers a new and higher level of security and agency. For this process, in which development is based on uncertainty and conflict, there are social structures or institutions, such as the family, parents, and teachers, which provide emotional support for this process, helping individuals progress from stage to stage and develop.

The fact that development takes place in such a conflict-ridden manner implies the possibility of non-development. As long as oppression and exploitation prevail in the various social formations, the all-encompassing competence of individual members of society is rendered impossible by the circumstances, it is prevented by the dominant authorities. Such impediments to achieving greater agency particularly affect women in our society, insofar as they are kept away, or keep themselves away, from the social process of production. Through various means such as bribery, diversion, repression, or compensation, they are persuaded to settle for lower levels of agency. This is particularly evident in all those spheres of social power where the conditions of agency take shape.

Before illustrating this connection with a few examples, I would like to formulate the following research guidelines from what has been said so far: in all contexts of oppression, the activities and attitudes of the oppressed must also be carefully analyzed. In addition to structural impediments, we should discover and identify conflict avoidance strategies and trace how alternative courses of action are missed through "seduction." Compensations, rewards, and concessions will likely guide the research paths taken. This applies both to historical research and to the analysis of individual socialization today.

Let us consider this through the example of the family in comparison to wage labour. Given that, under our current conditions, it is "oppressive" to be exclusively a mother and wife (for the well-known reason that women are not only excluded from any participation in social decision-making but also cannot provide for themselves, have no income of their own, cannot feed and clothe themselves, cannot live without their husbands' consent, etc.) we ask ourselves why women nevertheless "voluntarily" choose this condition, often knowing about this oppression and yet not preferring employment. This question does not seem so difficult to answer.

The advantages and disadvantages of being a wife and mother compared to wage labour are obvious. It can be small things; for example, the direct dependence on wage labour is not immediately and always apparent to the housewife. If she does not yet have children, she does not necessarily have to get up so early, she does not have to sell herself, she can dispose of her time as she wishes—at least, it seems as if she can. So, at some levels, she can choose a more immediately comfortable, more protected life over one that is more demanding but also more social, and, in that sense, a happier life. The difficulties of choosing the harder option are compounded by the fact that this emotional embeddedness appears as a seduction, socially supported as the dream of eternal love.

If learning and development are risks, and questioning old positions requires social security, then the learning and development opportunities for women in society as a whole look bleak. Positions of power and decision-making, indeed positions with reasonable prospects for advancement in wage labour, have not hitherto been envisaged for women in our society. In the social sphere, they therefore receive little emotional support for resolving conflicts assertively, walking tall. They will be outsiders. To ensure learning processes for women on a mass scale, different, hitherto unusual collectives are needed, a learning culture of their own. Here, the women's movement gains great significance; it becomes a necessity at every step in the learning that women must undertake to free themselves from social expectations.

Following the developmental condition outlined at the beginning, which concerned women being at the mercy of their own nature (contraception and baby formula that makes breast-feeding unnecessary), we now find the women's movement as a second necessary prerequisite for women's liberation. The women's movement and the women's cultures that have emerged within it provide individuals the opportunity to dissolve rigid structures within themselves and to take control of their own change.

I will now summarize these elements, which have been outlined here in a very brief form, in a different context, thereby arriving at an overall summary. The new question, under which I will further develop what has been said so far is.

What is the point of taking such a standpoint on women's activity in the face of their own oppression? In other words: who benefits from this analysis, which claims that women's oppression can only be grasped if one understands that women themselves have, step by step, consented to this practice of oppression? An initial answer: if we want to change something, if the women's movement wants to change and achieve something, we will find that our old personality structures stand in the way of change.

Consider, for example, the tremendous force with which most women cling to their private relationships and which they direct against themselves in every—inevitable—crisis, making these relationships more self-destructive than transformative. Furthermore, liberating change is challenged by a claim to effortlessness, which is usually already entrenched as part of the personality structure: expressed as a right to immediacy, to living well here and now, instead of the arduous efforts that every change requires. The private relationships mentioned above not only have self-destructive power, but they also occupy too much space in women's emotions. If we, as women, want to effect change, we must find the points of intervention that enable us to act ourselves. This means that, in order to act, we must change our own posture, and this is possible only through a change in our own personality structure. Why?

If we assume that talk of the oppression of women is not mere rhetoric, but that women actually live oppressed lives, that they must live their oppression as a daily practice, then we must also assume that the results of such a practice structure their personalities. If they are kept incapable in certain spheres, they can become capable of agency only by questioning parts of their own personalities. This, in turn, is a general characteristic of learning processes. In their attempt to become increasingly competent, increasingly independent, and to control more and more areas of their own lives, women will soon encounter spheres in which they cannot achieve the desired competence. In general, these are all spheres that secure the domination structures of society as a whole; for women, there are additional spheres of social intervention that hinder the process of individual socialization at a much earlier stage. The secret prohibitions on women's development, on "growing up," would drive individuals crazy, make them sick, and incapable of agency if they were conscious at every step that they are not allowed to become competent in these spheres.

It is true that enough people in our social conditions become crazy and ill, and this is especially true for women. However, those who do not go "crazy" but remain capable of agency at a limited level must, in their socialization process, reinterpret, repress, ignore, and exclude from their consciousness the individual spheres in which they are not allowed, or given the opportunity, to become competent. These misrepresentations form part of the personality structure. Such a structure can, for example, lead the excluded spheres to appear nonexistent, seem to have no emotional significance, occupy no place in women's feelings, and be perceived as boring.

If women want to change the conditions and relations under which they suffer, they must rebuild the spheres in which they have acquiesced to their incompetence into their own personalities, perceive things differently, that is, they must also change their feelings. This is a process of uncertainty, of particularly crisis-like proportions, a crisis that cannot be endured alone. It can only be overcome if there is some kind of security and support somewhere.[5]

And this brings me to my conclusion. If social support is not provided—and it undoubtedly is not—then, one might argue, political organizations and groups, therefore, a collective, are sufficient. I would like to argue here that this is not sufficient for women, because in this process of reorganizing their own feelings, the crisis-ridden transition from previous life structures to new ones, the men with whom women are, or would be, in these collectives and organizations introduce an additional element of tension that prevents reorientation. After all, men are also beneficiaries of these previously established personality structures. They cannot, therefore, offer unbiased support when women, for example, detach themselves from the absolute necessity of having a "personal relationship" that takes precedence over all other social activities, when they attach less importance to the family, when they want to have a say in decision-making and raise their voices. Enabling and implementing these processes of change is the historical right and necessity of the women's movement.

Notes

1 Editors' Note: The original essay was published as Frigga Haug, "Opfer oder Täter? Über das Verhalten von Frauen," *Das Argument*, no. 123 (1980): 643–649. *Opfer oder Täter?* It was previously translated by Rodney Livingston as "Victims or Culprits?" and published in *Beyond Female Masochism: Memory-Work and Politics* (Verso). For this publication, in consultation with Frigga Haug, we have decided to retranslate the text. The most significant change concerns the rendering of *Täter*—previously translated as *culprits*—as *agents*. Haug rejects the translation of *Täter* as culprits because, as its root *culpa* demonstrates, it connotes guilt, fault, or blame. While alternatives such as *maker* or *perpetrator* might also convey the meaning of *Täter*, the term *agent* best captures Haug's intended meaning and preserves its conceptual contrast with *Opfer* (victim). For further discussion, see the interview we conducted with Frigga Haug included in this volume.

2 In 2008, the year this text is reissued, marks the 100th anniversary of Simone de Beauvoir's birth. She is celebrated in the media as the starting point of intellectual feminism. Praised as a guiding maxim is the poor German translation of "On ne naît pas femme, on le deviant" as "We are not born as women, we are made into them." Misinterpreted in this way, it became a cornerstone of the discourse of victimhood within the women's movement.

3 Évelyne Sullerot (ed.), *Die Wirklichkeit der Frau* (Steinhausen, 1979). Translator's Note: Evelyne Sullerot was a prominent French feminist thinker, sociologist, and author known for her work on the *condition féminine* (the female condition) and the history of women's work, one of her most seminal notable texts being, *La Presse Féminine* (1963),

which is a survey and history of women's press. She was a leading figure in French feminist studies and held various international consultancies, including roles with the European Economic Community and the United Nations.

4 Klaus Holzkamp, *Zur kritisch-psychologischen Theorie der Subjektivität I & II*, Forum Kritische Psychologie 4 and 5 Argument-Sonderband 34 and 41 (Argument, 1979), Ute Holzkamp-Osterkamp, *Erkenntnis, Emotionalität und Handlungsfähigkeit*, Forum Kritische Psychologie 3, Argument-Sonderband 28 (Argument, 1978), Ute Holzkamp-Osterkamp, *Die Besonderheit menschlicher Bedürfnisse – Problematik und Erkenntnisgehalt der Psychoanalyse* (Campus, 1976).

5 The arguments presented here were elaborated and supported by empirical research, published in Frigga Haug, ed., *Erziehung zur Weiblichkeit. Frauenformen*, Argument-Sonderband, no. 45 (Argument, 1981).

References

Haug, Frigga, ed. *Erziehung zur Weiblichkeit. Frauenformen.* Argument-Sonderband, no. 45. Argument, 1981.

Haug, Frigga. "Victims or Culprits?" In *Beyond Female Masochism: Memory-Work and Politics*. Translated by Rodney Livingston. Verso, 1992.

Holzkamp, Klaus. "Zur kritisch-psychologischen Theorie der Subjektivität I & II." Forum Kritische Psychologie 4 and 5, *Argument-Sonderband*, no. 34 and 41. Argument, 1979.

Holzkamp-Osterkamp, Ute. *Die Besonderheit menschlicher Bedürfnisse – Problematik und Erkenntnisgehalt der Psychoanalyse*. Campus, 1976.

Holzkamp-Osterkamp, Ute. *Erkenntnis, Emotionalität und Handlungsfähigkeit*. Forum Kritische Psychologie 3, *Argument-Sonderband*, no. 28. Argument, 1978.

Sullerot, Évelyne. *Die Wirklichkeit der Frau*. Steinhausen, 1979.

Chapter 8

The Practice of Critique[1]

Frigga Haug

The suggestion to discuss the possibility and practice of critique in research and politics, which seemed to me to be a task, irritated me and forced me to explore further, walking as if on a patchwork quilt. Until then, I had readily assumed that the historical-critical method I had committed myself to was the only way to conduct research and that such a scientific foundation was essential for politics. But then I remembered an initially puzzling experience I had with my students. I taught at a "second-chance" university, an institution where the majority of students were working professionals who had gained admission not through a high school diploma, but through an exam after completing their professional training. I had created a seminar plan for them in which their experiences from "work" would be the starting point for demonstrating the usefulness of abstraction and conceptual penetration, using this as a new basis for lasting change. In short, I had set myself the high goal of making science accessible to them as something useful, even necessary, as a tool for understanding their lives; not for memorizing all kinds of abstractions to advance their careers, but as a way to penetrate the problems of capitalist societies in such a way that an alternative society would become visible as a perspective. I wanted to do this in a way that would help them realize that their work experience is a great foundation, not something contemptible, merely inadequate. In short, my ideas of teaching sociology and social psychology were quite extensively geared toward the education of the whole person. In this way, I wanted to use *the critique of political economy* in my teaching and, at the same time, explore a viable path to developing enthusiasm for science with these working students, more profoundly than with those who, coming out of high school, had no real-life experience and were expected to take on higher positions if they were successful, rather than those at the bottom. In short, I wanted to realize the left-wing dream of Rosa Luxemburg, that the problem of knowledgeable rulers and ignorant ruled could be shifted so that "everyone learns to take over the government."

That was in the late 1970s, more than ten years after 1968, the symbolic year of student rebellion. Apolitical calm had returned to the universities, and the teaching staff had been largely purged of Marxists. I was one of the Marxist who could no longer get a professorship at a regular university, but with the support of students and some teachers, I was able to become an assistant at a second-chance university,

DOI: 10.4324/9781003480143-8

founded in 1948 as the Academy for Public Economy. I was determined to use the situation as an opportunity, to think of these students as world changers, with whom the critique of political economy would fall on fertile ground, and who could simultaneously acquire scientific methods, theoretical critique, and social analysis.

Critique was such a natural foundation, doubt such an essential element of life, that I assumed that everyone was eager to move to critique after a phase of acquiring information and knowledge. But it was precisely at this early point in the teaching-learning drama that the flow of movement came to a half. The students were united in their resistance to using critique as a weapon, as something constructive and productive, let alone learning it beforehand. Some left the seminar, others went on standby. And after a period of astonishment and helplessness, I realized that I had to start all over again. I set aside all my carefully laid plans to incorporate work experience in such a way that it could be used to support historical-critical work and thus scientific insight. The question of critique itself had to take center stage. But how, if it was considered taboo?

During that semester, the students' refusal taught me a lot about myself, my thinking which was full of unexamined assumptions, about teaching, about learning, and, above all, it gave me a brief overview of the enormity of the unthought and unexplored wasteland that lay before me. It began with my assumption, based on a self-evident prejudice, that work experience was necessarily positive, something that second-chance students had over high school students. So I had blindly dismissed the fact that it is the experiences of waged labour that, through multiple forms of alienation, make life unbearable, make people sick, and shorten their lives. The experiences I wanted to draw on were not particularly fascinating for the students, but rather precisely what they wanted to leave behind. But the sting remained that experience, what was lived in sensual practical activity, must be the essential starting point for knowledge.

My new approach was to make not the experience of work (which, against my better judgment, I stubbornly regarded exclusively as waged labour) but rather the experience of critique the new starting point. The students wrote down memories and scenes of their experiences of critique. This move was the key to unlocking a vast treasure trove of experiences, suffering, feelings, disturbances, and pain. Critique was consistently a negative act inflicted on you by others. Critique was devaluation, non-recognition, destruction, rejection, withdrawal of love and friendship—in all areas, whether at home, at school, in training, or in everyday work, it was the weapon against the possibility of feeling at home in life, of being liked, supported, and wanted. All the available words, and there were more and more of them, the stream of remembered bad experiences became ever more abundant, were written down and showed that, against such an arsenal of defenses, it was unthinkable to use critique productively as a subject of teaching, let alone to consider the destruction of the familiar and the old as a possibility for new construction, for affirmative alternatives. I learned that in my initial approach, I even wanted to expect the students to become the agents of critique themselves, not only its victims.

The question had to be postponed once again. What was sought now was a positive experience with critique. A formulation had to be developed in such a way that the intended approach was based on common sense, that is, on what every person has despite all the burying, distortions, superstitions, and opinions. The discussion with the students plunged me into further abysses. In short, they did not want any critique at all, neither to experience nor exercise it, but rather praise and, in the context of wage labour, a working atmosphere in which flowers and birthday wishes from above demonstrate that you are respected as part of the workforce. They proved receptive to simple strategies for creating a feel-good atmosphere, the kind that are offered at every corner, which I, in turn, had learned to critique as a means of class struggle. In this way, it was clearly not possible to draw on experience. When you find yourself at a dead end, it is wise to choose a different path.

Hence, I changed track and examined how Marx dealt with the experiences of workers in his *Critique of Political Economy*. The first volume of *Capital* contains plenty experiences of labour—especially in the chapters on manufacturing, machinery, and large-scale industry—with detailed descriptions, particularly in footnotes, of labour activities and the misery in factories, all of which serve to sharpen the standpoint of critique. But they are not written by the workers, rather, within the horizon of a society without exploitation, they critically look at conditions in these areas from the standpoint of the development of productive forces. At the same time, it is quite obvious that Marx represents the workers' point of view, evaluates the reports of factory inspectors, and accurately records their resistance. How does learning from experience and dealing with experiences of labour factor into his critique?

There is, in fact, a document in which Marx addresses this question and uses a tool familiar to us: *The Workers' Questionnaire*.[2] This comprises 100 questions for workers, which were to be answered in writing and in detail. Twenty-five thousand copies were distributed in France, printed in *Revue Socialiste* magazine, and translated into English and German. It seems hardly surprising to me that there was no significant response, no subsequent major evaluation, and no multi-volume publication. Answering the questions would have overwhelmed any individual, required some of them to do their own research, and, in any case, taken many hours. What is remarkable, however, is that Marx breaks with conventional social surveys, to the extent that they even existed, and calls on workers themselves to become researchers in their own cause. Looking back, it is downright amusing to see how Marx puts together the individual elements of the theory of surplus value and gradually brings them into conscious experience. Most of the questions are still suitable for training seminars in which participants are not simply informed and instructed, but rather their knowledge is brought to consciousness and can be collectively assembled into complex theorems, such as the theory of surplus value.[3] The questionnaire is also a careful elaboration of Marx's famous earlier statement: "It will then become evident that the world has long dreamed of possessing something of which it has only to be conscious of in order to possess it in reality."[4] Dull suffering is replaced by a consciousness of the situation, which is a prerequisite for the ability to act, because concrete knowledge about disorders, discomfort, and illness provides the opportunity to intervene.

From this ever-surprising testimony, I turn to Marx and his "Theses on Feuerbach," in which he outlines the main points of his overall project, the great *critique of political economy*, in a concise manner:

> First thesis: "The chief defect of all previous materialism (that of Feuerbach included) is that things [Gegenstand], reality, sensuousness are conceived only in the form of the object, or of contemplation, but not as sensuous human activity, practice, not subjectively....Hence he does not grasp the significance of 'revolutionary', of 'practical-critical', activity."
>
> Third thesis: "The coincidence of the changing of circumstances and of human activity or self-change can be conceived and rationally understood only as *revolutionary practice.*"[5]

My politicization as part of the first generation of students who began to read Marx seriously—in the mid-1960s—took place in such a way that we read the words chosen in the "Theses on Feuerbach" as if they were foreign words, even when they seemed commonplace, and did not truly understand them. This applied to everything essential: materialism, object, reality, sensuality, the form of the object or perception, sensuous human activity, practice, subjective, practical-critical activity, self-transformation, revolutionary practice. Even today, 50 years later, I discover something new every time I read it, whole worlds of unnoticed analysis and critique, and I assume that this is a fairly common experience, one that warrants careful analysis and its own autobiographical, historical-critical approach. Although I studied in an environment drawn to Marx, the Feuerbach theses remained silent—or rather, we spoke differently with the same words.

I was one of the first sociology students at the Freie Universität Berlin and learned that this was the science of society, its fundamental question being: How is society possible? Until then, it was considered—in a way that is completely incomprehensible to later generations—that uttering the word "society" implied bad company: a proximity to communism and materialism, a crossing of the border into a forbidden zone, on the impossibility of which the Freie Universität was founded (where I immediately became politically active in the student parliament). In sociology, we had to deal with abstractions in a challenging and new way, with structure, institutions, classes, and strata; our student politics were directed against our origins in fascism, and our commitment was to everything that opposed war and aimed at preventing it. The distance between the new things we had to learn and our individual pasts initially prevented us from engaging with ourselves, at least not publicly. The sensuous, the subjective, and the associated practices, self-transformation, suddenly found themselves on the side of the old that was to be avoided; thus the "revolutionary" that inspired us as students amid change became an abstract, distant goal and, as such, an act that took place somewhere in the past, in history, and in the present, in distant lands. It would concern us only if we became followers in bloody, dangerous activities, as the cult films of the time (such as *Maria and Maria*) suggested. The key to our lives, "The coincidence of the changing of circumstances and of human activity or self-change can be conceived and rationally understood only as revolutionary practice," could be tucked away unheard into the ever-growing reservoir of the "non-understandable" that accompanies studying.[6]

Critique of Capitalism, Women's History, and Everyday Research

However, we studied Marx's *Capital* in our reading groups, which gathered around the journal, *The Argument*. Critiques of capitalism grew alongside critiques of fascism and war, and we became part of the left—socialists with a proud sense of belonging and no awareness of what society in the past and present had to do with our constitution and that of "others." We did not even ask how the state, capitalism, and ideology, assumed to be external conditions, penetrate the inner workings of each individual, how we, as human beings, became what we are today, and where we are headed.

That was the end of the 1960s; the student movement's protests affected everyday life, habits, norms, and morals, yet overlooked women's inequality, even in the midst of revolt. The women's movement, which began shortly thereafter, only logically opposed this through self-consciousness groups. Large gatherings were held where one woman after another stood up and recounted their personal experiences of oppression, disrespect, and cruelty. This practice seemed both right and appropriate—how else could women's history emerge from the sidelines of the undocumented into general consciousness? —yet it also seemed misguided, because while many wanted to speak, the many who were waiting for their turn were needed as listeners, not speakers, and the constant repetition soon dulled rather than led to understanding.

In many countries and their universities, the study of women's history was taken up and given encyclopedic status as a separate discipline and subject. However, something was still emphatically missing—that which is contained in the third Feuerbach thesis, the fulfilment of what only during my university years suddenly became legible as a promise: that self-transformation and the transformation of conditions coincide in revolutionary practice. The preoccupation with oneself had to shift from what carried the stench of affluent women who have time, money, and nothing else to do, to becoming integrally connected with critical and revolutionary practice that changes society. The paralyzing exclusion of one by the other (the either/or of studying oneself or the conditions) had gained momentum through the close union of the mutually exclusive. In revolutionary change, both sides are in motion: the critical individuals and the relations that need to be changed; this necessitates continuous critical work, self-reflection, the study of power relations, and thus a wholehearted commitment to change. The call to change has shifted from being a moral imperative demanding obedience and docility to one that, conversely, seems to command disobedience and permanent rebellion against authority. For some, anti-authoritarian education became the order of the day, while others impatiently understood it as a call to join revolutions somewhere in the world with all their passion or to instigate them in their own cities, thus also understanding the word "revolution" as a kind of foreign religion that one had to profess in order to then take action: the fight against external enemies. They received all the media attention and thus garnered more supporters, while the Marxist feminists, moving tentatively, were unable, or unwilling, go along with the rapidly growing tide of feminists.

Women also Make Their Own History

Feminist Marxists who emerged from the student movement began to examine how the subjugation of the female sex (its "world-historic defeat," as Engels puts it in *Origin of the Family*[7]) should not simply be thought of and understood as an overpowering of women by a male conspiracy but rather requires examining how control over female bodies (labour power and sexuality) receives the consent of the oppressed, who usually produce and reproduce it throughout their lives. The title of an early book in the women's movement, *We Are Not Born as Girls, We Are Made So*, rightly protests against the idea of a predetermined female nature, but it remains trapped within the notion of men as enemies and women as their victims.[8] The debate about victims and agents that began in the 1970s[9] calls for the difficult task of searching for the "enemies" within oneself, that is exploring the co-production of one's own oppression in capitalist conditions. Marx and Lassalle, albeit in different ways, also express as fundamental the idea that people create their own history, even if not of their own free will.[10] As Rosa Luxemburg points out:

> At first glance, everything good and evil, the happiness and the misery of peoples, is the work of individual rulers or great men. In reality, the people, the nameless masses themselves, make their fate, happiness, and woe.[11]

The development of memory work, with which most people in this room are probably familiar, is necessary because it proved to be the most convincing method during my teaching and lectures in Denmark (including in Roskilde), not least because it directly involves all participants, whether teachers or students, in research about themselves without requiring embarrassing self-disclosure, while simultaneously adding knowledge to the subject at hand. Memory work, just like Marx's workers' questionnaires, draws on experience from one's past (or even present) and thus assumes that each one knows more about herself than she thinks. This knowledge must be brought to the fore and conceptualized, that is, freed from dull heaviness and painful forgetfulness into conscious knowledge and thereby made available to those involved. The analysis of relations is supplemented by the microscopic analysis of individual biographies carried out by the actors themselves. The historical-critical method for this is precisely *memory work* and upholds Brecht's exhortation to live in the third person.[12] This also means overcoming the inconsequential morality of the usual discourse on self-transformation in favor of an imperative for self-reflection and, in turn, reporting on oneself in remembering and writing as if one were a stranger that one gets to know. This sharpens the eye, enforces accountability, distinguishes between what is essential and what is unnecessary, can be incorruptible, and can detect and decisively reject complicity with domination.

The study of Antonio Gramsci's *Prison Notebooks* was essential for this constant change.[13] He makes a series of suggestions that seem directly intended for the process of memory work. He recommends suggestions for a *philosophy of praxis* that incorporates each individual's worldview. Gramsci succinctly demonstrates that "human beings," as social beings must create an *inventory* of themselves in order to continuously strive to change themselves. This task is not just psychological, but above all political, because it necessarily includes shaping society. "So one could say that each one of us changes himself, modifies himself to the extent that he changes and modifies the complex relations of which he is the hub."[14] This presupposes that

> [i]t is not enough to know the ensemble of relations as they exist at any given time as a given system. They must be known genetically, in the movement of their formation. For each individual is the synthesis not only of existing relations, but of the history of these relations. He is a precis of all the past.[15]

In his *Introduction to the Study of Philosophy*, Gramsci takes up these ideas and at the same time summarizes other pioneering elements.[16] Notably, he writes from a perspective that begins in a somewhat negative way, assuming that the current state of affairs is *not yet* complete.

> When one's conception of the world is not critical and coherent but disjointed and episodic, one belongs simultaneously to a multiplicity of mass human groups. The personality is strangely composite: it contains Stone Age elements and principles of a more advanced science, prejudices from all past phases of history at the local level and intuitions of a future philosophy which will be that of a human race united the world over. To criticise one's own conception of the world means therefore to make it a coherent unity and to raise it to the level reached by the most advanced thought in the world. It therefore also means criticism of all previous philosophy, in so far as this has left stratified deposits in popular philosophy. The starting-point of critical elaboration is the consciousness of what one really is, and is 'knowing thy self' as a product of the historical process to date which has deposited in you an infinity of traces, without leaving an inventory.[17]

It remains to be explained why such proposals made by Gramsci eight decades ago fell largely unheard and into oblivion, despite an excellent translation of his writings in the 1980s. Equally strange is that post-Marxist gender research proclaims as brand new the idea that women are a product of social construction, using this to disarticulate feminist-Marxist research by removing woman as a solidarity-based subject and rejecting the work on the basis of its own coherence in favor of recognizing internal diversity.

Back to memory work. Its goal is the ability to act with solidarity in political action and critical insight. It relies on collective self-determination, on learning with the prerequisites of politics from below, on the desire for self-development and self-affirmation. By striving to raise consciousness among the participants, like in Marx's questionnaire, and by making them conscious of what they already know, memory work deals with language and meanings. It finds itself in constant close combat with everyday language, which is occupied by dominant ideology and opinion, by habits, and by what is considered to be true. Memory work bets on the good life, even though this has long had a sour aftertaste or been seized to the point of corruption. In a sense, it bets on the solidarity of common sense in each individual and its reassurance within a collective that shares the same goal of replacing generally avoidable misfortune with possible happiness.

Self-Critique

In memory work, self-critique is an elementary dimension of knowledge. One person guides the process, but they themselves, like the others, are both researcher and object of research, both subject and object. She alone knows her experiences in such detail that comparisons can be made, mistakes and errors can be discussed, and general prejudices can be revealed that, in terms of political correctness, one would not have suspected in oneself. In the search for how the recognized relations reproduce themselves, and are thus reproduced by everyone, doubt becomes productive critique and self-critique a source of further knowledge and, at the same time, compelling in itself.[18]

After posing the troubling question of whether, as a committed researcher from below and representative of self-determination, one can justify a leader in collective memory work, this doubt had to be extended to the teacher itself. We had criticized the school as an institution to such an extent that it had to be rejected as an one that prevents learning,[19] we rejected the specification of learning content through curricula, and, had taken our doubts so far that even regarding the problem of learning processes, the autonomous individual alone could be consider the originator—until I was able to radicalize the question: Why do students need teachers at all?—After further prolonged doubt, I returned to the original paradigm: experience. My conclusion was that teachers are necessary to lead experiences into crisis, to initiate unlearning, to interrupt the constant reproduction of domination through habits. This work remains controversial in critical psychology to this day and requires further development. Brecht, who, as I read much later, describes such a process as putting "opinions…into a state of crisis."[20] His method, which can be called scientific, can be extracted from numerous notes and elaborate prose.[21] It consists in not presenting a view, a world view, a conviction, or even an opinion that is wholly shallow as false, not to refute it; but rather, in examining how it comes about, what experiences it bundles, which allowed for the existing judgment, to seek out a counter-experience (at the same level be it analytical or abstract), and in doing so to bring about a crisis that makes one's own investigation and reflection mandatory to arrive at a new judgment. In short, Brecht gives advice for constant self-reflection.

Perceiving the world self-critically unleashes both imagination and learning processes.

The Productivity of Critique

However, what exactly does critique mean, or what do we mean when we speak of critique? Until this point, it has been tacitly assumed that critique based on accusation, indictment, and condemnation, which students apparently rejected at the beginning of their academic studies, is not what should be demonstrated as productive for research and knowledge when considering its potential for research and practice. At this point, we cannot engage in a treatise on the thinking about critique, use of language, origin, etc., but rather, for our questions in labour research, pedagogy, women's studies, and psychology, we ruthlessly draw from the pool of historical knowledge what we find fruitful for further work.[22] Here, I briefly mentioned Marx's inclusion of workers for self-research and Gramsci for memory work and then immediately turned to the empirical evidence of some of our practices.

However, there is more to learn from Marx about critique than from his questionnaire. He critiques subjects, relations, ideas, science, theories, and behavior—above all, he examines inversions, how the active, including those who act, come to assume the status of objects. How labour takes on the form of value, how what people do confronts them as something that can be bought and sold on the marketplace, and how this then continues to determine society, as if the workers had nothing to do with it. In Marx, one can study how what people usually do to preserve themselves needfully and pleasurably—to reproduce themselves precariously and pleasurably—organizes upbringing, without their knowing it, in determinate forms (such as the family), how all of this enters into the form of religion, into morality and values.[23] One's activities become alien powers that control people, who in turn submit to them. Or, in other words, Marx examines self-contradictions that take on various forms. He does not examine individual phenomena in terms of their opposites, such as friends versus enemies, good versus evil, but rather the genesis of a practice, the form it takes, and how that form determines perception. The entire undertaking is one of critique, which examines, distinguishes, judges, and places things in new contexts with the aim of gaining clarity about human relationships and relations so that the possibility of non-domination can be a perspective and guideline for action.

Critique is of particular interest here as a method of discovery. Just as Socrates used the art of discovery to suggest talking through what has become entrenched, of liquefying views that have become rigid to arrive at an immanent sublation (dialogical midwifery), we—in *The Automation and Qualification Project*—employed this well-known method and invented, for example, in a study on the computerization of offices, *the contradiction-led group interview.*[24] The aim was to identify practical experiences in learning the new technology, although we knew that the introductory courses were largely attended only by men, and that women, who were the majority in administration and public service, immediately took over tasks such as making the workplace comfortable, preparing coffee, and running numerous errands. At the same time, we recognized that approaching this learning as equals, so to speak, would not be easy, as long as the new devices were perceived primarily as technical and not mere writing implements. All the prejudices about technical aptitude and women's innate, orderly diligence would simultaneously come into a forceful clash. However, we also knew that the acceptance of the old division of labour in new relations also required the consent of the workers.

At first, nothing exciting happened in the group discussion; individuals tediously repeated how they had taken on certain tasks, as if this had been of their own free will. The challenge now was to organize the self-contradictions, and we found that the best approach was to choose a widely experienced yet rarely discussed contradiction as a source of knowledge. This was gender relations, both in the workplace and elsewhere. In our industrialized capitalist countries, there is a general consensus that the sexes should have equal rights and responsibilities, equal recognition, and indeed equal wages; any inequalities are seen as asynchronicities that require reform. At the same time, everyone knows that things are different in practice. In the case of learning new technology, it would suffice to invoke equality as a contradiction and counterfactually assert a corresponding practice of learning. In our case, the previous tenacious harmony in the conversation was immediately broken by a heated discussion in which one gender accused the other of countless mistakes, omissions, neglect, repression, and so on—so that the practice of how it was learned (or not learned), what disruptions occurred, etc., could be clearly identified. We also learned how many crises it takes to bring about real changes in old divisions of labour and associated habits.

Although I do not know whether rapidly changing technology will continue to reproduce old divisions of labour, I have chosen the example of office computerization to demonstrate the overall strategic relevance of gender relations—which Marx also mentioned but did not carefully develop for the problem of critique, knowledge, and politics—in order to open them up for discussion. Several years ago, I wrote the following without receiving any significant response,

> Gender relations should be understood as complex praxis relations. Their analysis considers both the formation of the actors and the reproduction of society as a whole. They can be understood as 'fundamental regulatory relations in all social formations': they cross through (and are in turn central to) questions of division of labour, domination, exploitation, ideology, politics, law, religion, morality,

> sexuality, body and senses, language; indeed, basically no area can be meaningfully examined without exploring how gender relations are formed and shaped.[25]

The oppression of women is, therefore, embedded in the foundation of the capitalist mode of production, like the exploitation and incorporation of traditional modes of production. These extremely crisis-ridden capitalist relations of production deepen divisions in society, create an army of superfluous people, and exhaust resources. Capitalism thrives on the intertwining of large divisions of labour (city and country, head and hand, men's and women's labour) and overcoming it requires the dissolution of this interaction, or rather the analysis and processing of its impact on culture, politics, wage labour, and reproduction. Years later, in 2008, I proposed a project for this process, intended to be both politically oriented and to promote knowledge acquisition, which I called the *four-in-one perspective*.[26] It begins with the disposal of time as the basis of all domination and arranges the respective activities in a different order from the usual. Each activity should be equal to every other. Each should be supported by all. Each should be granted as a right and become the responsibility of everyone. However, this new arrangement changes the significance of each type of activity for society as a whole as well as for individuals. The transformation of living conditions and self-transformation coincide, so that the demand for everyone to participate in shaping society does not remain a mere phrase but becomes a social necessity.

One of the prerequisites and, at the same time, one of the ever-changing results, is that critical thinking cannot develop through simple negation, nor through mere opposition, nor by replacing obedience with disobedience, nor by seizing power to escape subjugation, nor by rising to the top to escape being at the bottom, but through the explication of self-contradiction. Obstacles, conscious resistance, crises, and wars pile up along this path. The opposing forces are present both in existing structures and state-supported economic interests, as well as within individuals themselves. This applies particularly to women in their natural divisions of labour as well as in the corresponding state-backed ideologies, values, morals, and protective dependency structures. A continuous study of the balance of power is essential, and accordingly, the generalization of scientific research thinking and language politics is also a major task of critical thinking. Confronting the various forces that individually determine events, sometimes more, sometimes less dominantly, would only forge the shackles more firmly; they must be wrestled with simultaneously, which requires a different division of labour between men and women regarding responsibility for others, time for self-development, and the formation of politics.

What I refer to as the domination knot is the intertwining of different threads that support and sustain each other, several of which are invisible but whose interconnectedness keeps capitalist society running. Intertwined in this knot are: the profit-driven actions of capital that incorporate living labour in the form of wage labour, thereby always further developing the productive forces, thereby depleting and cutting back on labour, which is its source—this is already a complex dialectical connection.

Then there are the invisible, unspoken, and historyless deeds that are all necessary to restore the lives of people and the nature surrounding them. These form a thread, have a different temporal logic, are difficult to rationalize—that is, make more efficient and faster—in order to be profitable: the different forms of the loving mother, the heroic nurse, the volunteer charity worker, and the environmentalist are just as well-known as the catastrophes that attack people from behind, from the brutalization and degeneration of entire generations and sections of the population to the uninhabitability of the earth. Many of these activities remain invisible—and many have been transformed into wage labour in developed capitalist countries, where they have a tolerated, poor, and poorly paid reputation.

Within this interlocking, the neglect of people themselves as human beings goes almost unmentioned—development is elitist, something that only the rich can afford, while the urge to develop what is humanly possible is stifled in the consumer frenzy, which is also a basis for growth, consumption, etc., and it also goes unnoticed that people are kept subaltern in immaturity regarding the shaping of society—what we call politics. These four threads are intricately interwoven, secured, and developed and can be found in our habits, actions, morals, hopes, desires, and common sense. Acts of change are themselves the common revolutionary practice that seemed so alien in the Feuerbach theses. Despite all skepticism about the development of socially productive forces in natural science, technology, and biology, there remains a categorical necessity to constantly improve living conditions for everyone, that is, to exercise critique as a driving force for change.

Notes

1 This text was delivered as a speech by Frigga Haug upon receiving an honorary doctorate degree from the University of Roskilde in September 2016.

2 Karl Marx, "Fragebogen für Arbeiter," *Marx Engels Werke Band 19* (Dietz, 1987), 230–237; Karl Marx, "Workers' Questionnaire," *Marx and Engels Collected Works, Volume 24: Marx and Engels 1874–83* (International Publishers, 1976), 328–334.

3 For example, questions 15 and 16, 27 – conditions at the workplace and everything that goes with them, and their impact on health; in II: 11, 14, 16, loss of time, children's school and learning content; in III 3 and 4, penalties for breach of contract 11, 12, 13 for labour performed in advance, 24, necessary items and their prices, 27–29, 30, economic fluctuations without such fluctuations in wage relations, 35 prospects for retirement, IV strikes, servants of wage masters, profit sharing.

4 Karl Marx, "Brief an Arnold Ruge," *Marx Engels Werke Band 1* (Dietz, 1981), 343–346, 347; Karl Marx, "Letters from the Deutsch-französische Jahrbücher. Letter to Arnold Ruge," *Marx and Engels Collected Works, Volume 3: Karl Marx March 1843-August 1844* (International Publishers, 1975), 141–145, 144.

5 Karl Marx, "Thesen über Feuerbach," *Marx Engels Werke Band 3* (Dietz, 1969), 5–7, 5–6; Karl Marx, "Theses on Feuerbach," *Marx and Engels Collected Works, Volume 5: Marx and Engels 1845–47* (International Publishers, 1976), 3–5, 3–4.

6 Marx, "Thesen über Feuerbach," 6; Marx, "Theses on Feuerbach," 4.

7 Friedrich Engels, "Der Ursprung der Familie, des Privateigentums und des Staats," *Marx Engels Werke Band 21* (Dietz 1962), 25–173, 61; Frederick Engels, "The Origin of the

Family, Private Property and the State," *Marx and Engels Collected Works, Volume 26: Engels 1882–89* (International Publishers, 1976), 126–276, 165.
8 Ursula Scheu, *Wir werden nicht als Mädchen geboren - wir werden dazu gemacht: Zur frühkindlichen Erziehung in unserer Gesellschaft* (Fischer, 1997).
9 Frigga Haug, "Opfer oder Täter?: Über das Verhalten von Frauen," *Das Argument*, no. 123 (1980): 643–649; For English, see "Victims or Agents," in this volume.
10 Sickingen debate: Luxemburg sums up the Sickingen debate between Marx and Lassalle as follows: "What is being fought out here between Lassalle and Marx is [...] not the opposition between the idealist and materialist conception of history, but rather a difference within the latter, which the two grasp at different moments. People make their own history, but they do not make it of their own free will, said Marx and Engels, defending their life's work, the lawful materialist explanation of history. People do not make history of their own free will, but they make it themselves, emphasized Lassalle, defending his life's work, the 'individual decision,' the 'bold deed.'" See Rosa Luxemburg, *Gesammelte Werke Band 1.2: 1893 bis 1905* (Dietz, 2003), 155.
11 Rosa Luxemburg, *Gesammelte Werke Band 4: August 1914 bis Januar 1919* (Dietz, 2003), 206.
12 Frigga Haug, *Erinnerungsarbeit* (Argument-Verlag, 1990).
13 Antonio Gramsci, "Philosophie der Praxis," *Gefängnishefte*, ed. Klaus Bochmann, Haug Wolfgang Fritz (Argument, 1994); Antonio Gramsci, *Selections from the Prison Notebooks* (International Publishers, 1971).
14 Gramsci, "Philosophie der Praxis," Band 6, Heft 10, § 54, 1348; Gramsci, *Selections from the Prison Notebooks*, 352.
15 Gramsci, "Philosophie der Praxis," Band 6, Heft 10, § 54, 1348; Gramsci, *Selections from the Prison Notebooks*, 353.
16 Gramsci, "Philosophie der Praxis," Heft 11, 1364–1493; Gramsci, *Selections from the Prison Notebooks*, 321–377.
17 Gramsci, "Philosophie der Praxis," Heft 12, § 12, 1376; Gramsci, *Selections from the Prison Notebooks*, 324.
18 The misunderstood emancipation and defense of the women's movement against feminism under the Gramscian motto of inventory without reservation is further explored in my book, *Der im Gehen erkundete Weg. Marxismus-Feminismus* [The Path Explored while Walking-Marxism-Feminism] (Argument Verlag, 2015).
19 Klaus Holzkamp, *Lernen: Subjektwissenschaftliche Grundlegung* [Learning: Subject Scientific Foundation] (Campus, 1995).
20 Berthold Brecht, "Dialektische Kritik," in *Schriften zur Politik und Gesellschaft*, Gesammelte Werke 20 (Suhrkamp, Frankfurt/M. 1967), 153; Bertolt Brecht, *Brecht on Art and Politics*, trans. Laura Bradley et al. (Bloomsbury Publishing, 2003), 104.
21 Brecht, "Dialektische Kritik," 153. See also Bertolt Brecht, *Me-ti. Buch der Wendungen* (Suhrkamp, 1983); Bertolt Brecht, *Me-ti: Book of Interventions in the Flow of Things* (Methuen Drama, 2016).
22 "Kritik" [Critique] in *Historisch-Kritisches Wörterbuch des Marxismus*, ed. Wolfang Fritz Haug, Frigga Haug, Peter Jehle and Wolfgang Küttler (Argument, 2012), 39–108.
23 Karl Marx and Friedrich Engels, "Die heilige Familie," *Marx Engels Werke Band 2* (Dietz, 1962), 3–224; Karl Marx and Frederick Engels, "The Holy Family," *Marx and Engels Collected Works, Volume 4: Marx and Engels 1844–45* (International Publishers, 1976), 5–294.
24 The 'Automation and Qualification' research project (PAQ) was launched at the (independent) Institute of Psychology at the Free University of Berlin in 1972 and lasted for 16 years, despite the scattered locations of the research group's members. See Frigga Haug, "The Journey of the 'Automation and Qualification' Project," *Marx and the*

Robots: Networked Production, AI and Human Labour, ed. Florian Butollo and Sabine Nuss and trans. Jan-Peter Herrmann with Nivene Raafat (Pluto Press, 2022), 67–85.

25 "Geschlechterverhältnisse" [Gender Relations] in *Historisch-Kritisches Wörterbuch des Marxismus*, ed. Wolfang Fritz Haug, Frigga Haug, Peter Jehle and Wolfgang Küttler (Argument, 2001), 493–531, 493.

26 Editors' Note: for more on this topic, see the essay, "Four-in-One-Perspective," in this volume.

References

Brecht, Bertolt. "Dialektische Kritik." In *Schriften zur Politik und Gesellschaft, Gesammelte Werke* 20. Suhrkamp, 1967.

Brecht, Bertolt. *Me-ti. Buch der Wendungen.* Suhrkamp, 1983.

Brecht, Bertolt. *Brecht on Art and Politics.* Translated by Laura Bradley, Julian Preece, and Stephen Parker. Bloomsbury Publishing, 2003.

Brecht, Bertolt. *Me-ti: Book of Interventions in the Flow of Things*. Methuen Drama, 2016.

Engels, Friedrich. "Der Ursprung der Familie, des Privateigentums und des Staats." In *Marx Engels Werke Band 21*. Dietz, 1962.

Engels, Frederick. "The Origin of the Family, Private Property and the State." In *Marx and Engels Collected Works, Volume* 26: Engels 1882–89, 126–276. International Publishers, 1976.

Gramsci, Antonio. *Gefängnishefte.* Edited by Klaus Bochmann and Wolfgang Fritz Haug. Argument, 1994.

Gramsci, Antonio. *Selections from the Prison Notebooks*. International Publishers, 1971.

Haug, Frigga. "Opfer oder Täter? Über das Verhalten von Frauen." *Das Argument*, no. 123 (1980): 643–649.

Haug, Frigga. *Erinnerungsarbeit.* Argument Verlag, 1990.

Haug, Frigga. *Der im Gehen erkundete Weg. Marxismus-Feminismus.* Argument Verlag, 2015.

Haug, Frigga. "The Journey of the 'Automation and Qualification' Project." In *Marx and the Robots: Networked Production, AI and Human Labour*. Edited by Florian Butollo and Sabine Nuss and translated by Jan-Peter Herrmann and Nivene Raafat. Pluto Press, 2022.

Holzkamp, Klaus. *Lernen: Subjektwissenschaftliche Grundlegung*. Campus, 1995.

"Kritik." In *Historisch-Kritisches Wörterbuch des Marxismus*. Edited by Wolfgang Fritz Haug, Frigga Haug, Peter Jehle, and Wolfgang Küttler. Argument, 2012.

"Geschlechterverhältnisse." In *Historisch-Kritisches Wörterbuch des Marxismus*. Edited by Wolfgang Fritz Haug, Frigga Haug, Peter Jehle, and Wolfgang Küttler. Argument, 2001.

Luxemburg, Rosa. *Gesammelte Werke Band 1.2*: 1893 bis 1905. Dietz, 2003a.

Luxemburg, Rosa. *Gesammelte Werke Band 4*: August 1914 bis Januar 1919. Dietz, 2003b.

Marx, Karl. "Thesen über Feuerbach." *Marx Engels Werke* 3. Dietz, 1969.

Marx, Karl. "Letters from the Deutsch-französische Jahrbücher. Letter to Arnold Ruge." In *Marx and Engels Collected Works, Volume* 3*: Karl Marx March 1843–August 1844.* International Publishers, 1975.

Marx, Karl. "Workers' Questionnaire." In *Marx and Engels Collected Works, Volume 24: Marx and Engels 1874–83*. International Publishers, 1976a.

Marx, Karl. "Theses on Feuerbach." In *Marx and Engels Collected Works, Volume 5: Marx and Engels 1845–47*. International Publishers, 1976b.

Marx, Karl. "Brief an Arnold Ruge." *Marx Engels Werke* 1. Dietz, 1981.

Marx, Karl. "Fragebogen für Arbeiter." *Marx Engels Werke* 19 (Dietz 1987), 230–237.

Marx, Karl, and Friedrich Engels. "Die heilige Familie." *Marx Engels Werke Band 2.* Dietz 1962.

Marx, Karl, and Friedrich Engels. "The Holy Family." In *Marx and Engels Collected Works, Volume 4: Marx and Engels 1844–45*. International Publishers, 1976.

Scheu, Ursula. *Wir werden nicht als Mädchen geboren – wir werden dazu gemacht. Zur frühkindlichen Erziehung in unserer Gesellschaft*. Fischer, 1997.

Chapter 9

Feminist Work with Marx[1]

Frigga Haug

An exploration of the theoretical background of memory work cannot avoid a discussion of Marx. The aim is to work out what can be inherited from Marx, what aspects of his work need to be critically continued to be useful for a feminist project. This chapter, therefore, does not revisit the feminist dispute about Marx,[2] but intervenes at three points and draws lessons from Marx that I to consider to be very fruitful, even indispensable, for contemporary feminism. These are:

1 The significance of Marx's theses against Feuerbach for feminist research and the critique of bourgeois science;
2 The question of Marx's concept of labour, which, on the one hand, continues to determine feminist debates to this day and, on the other hand, should be more precisely recalled and defined for a discussion in the current "crisis of the working society"; and finally,
3 Marx's treatment of family and housework, which, in my opinion, accompanies the entire critique of political economy in a one-sided manner and therefore does not sufficiently articulate a critique of the capitalist social formation, even in its current form.

Marx and Labour

The initial feminist anger toward Marx, which ultimately led to a rejection of Marxist thinking, was not directed at the Feuerbach theses, whose significance for scientific feminism I found nowhere explained, but at his concept of labour and theories on the production of surplus value.

The accusation was that Marx had developed a concept of labour that excluded women and ultimately prevented him from recognizing women's oppression. The criticism focused on his view of the "dual character of labour." The idea that labour creates both use values and exchange values is central to his analysis of capitalism and its dynamics, as well as to his theory of revolution. A society that is driven by transforming living labour into dead labour (to speak in Marxian metaphors) and then giving dead labour power over living labour in the form of capital, machines, and factories will maneuver itself into catastrophe if

DOI: 10.4324/9781003480143-9

no radical intervention takes place. However, such a radical act would have to overthrow the fundamental structures of social regulation: profit as the driving force and, with it, the dominance of surplus value over living labour based on the division of labour and property. In his analysis of the dual character of labour, Marx focuses on wage labour as the determining factor in deforming life activity. A first revolutionary step would be the abolition of private ownership of the means of production. This argument resulted in the male worker, in his historical role as the breadwinner of the family, becoming the center of analysis, just as the labour movement became the subject of politics. Women's protests against this theoretical arrangement seem justified. For even if we agree that this situation is a creation of capitalist society and not simply of Marxist analysis, there is a remarkable emptiness and silence in his argument where women should have been discussed. The housework debate of the late 1960s and early 1970s, which in a sense continued on the internet, at least in the United States, into the late 1990s, extends this criticism of the focus on the male worker to a discussion of the validity of the Marx's theory of value in general.

The early discussion in feminism was sparked by the question of forgotten housework in Marx's theory of value. Following Mariarosa Dalla Costa (1973),[3] the theory of value is expanded to include housework, which is claimed to be "productive" because it reproduces labour power as a commodity in the form of personal services, thereby ensuring the increase of surplus value behind the back of industrial production. The role of woman is often made invisible in the form of *family work*. Women also produce more value than is necessary for their own reproduction, the free appropriation of which is incorporated into capital profit and is not taken into account by Marx. In this analysis, the family becomes a center of social production. *Housework* was also highlighted as a "blind spot in the critique of political economy."[4] What is even more serious for Werlhof, however, is that wage discrimination against women is actually justified because women create less value. This is explained by the fact that women reproduce men, but their own reproduction must be subtracted from their powers. In this respect, men were in fact more valuable for entrepreneurs, who with the purchase of male labour power also acquired an invisible and free share of *women's labour*. The neglect of the work done by women at home in the reproduction of labour power was bound to ignore an essential component of the surplus value appropriated by capitalists. If the secret of the commodity labour power was that it was able to produce more than it needed for its own reproduction, then this had to apply to women as well, and it had to be determined how this additional labour power also entered into the capitalist commodity-production.[5] One practical consequence of such analyses was the demand for wages for *housework*; another was to simply abolish this sphere of unpaid female labour. Perhaps one cannot deny some plausibility to such arguments, but what seems problematic to me is that these discussions were largely purely academic and inconsequential, since the passion that went into the debate about the value of domestic labour found little equivalent in a corresponding political strategy.

On the other hand, the argument that housework is also productive and should therefore be socially recognized and paid for in the same way as wage labour, which was also explicitly stated in the housework debate, had political influence. More conservative parties in Germany adopted the demand for wages for housework, as it could simultaneously serve to uphold the "value of the family" and gain approval for women's decision not to work, which seemed increasingly advantageous in the face of raising unemployment.[6] With the justified protest against the disregard for domestic work through its unceremonious inscription on a kind of equal footing with wage labour, almost everything that the women's movement had begun to fight for was abandoned: the critique of the form of the family, the sexual division of labour, the alienated form of wage labour, and capitalism. The claim that housework was also productive could, if only through a sleight of hand, cover up the flaw of a form of division of labour that denied women, as soon as they engaged in housework exclusively, the possibility of even existing without a male breadwinner.

The debate continued as a feminist one, primarily in the United States. In their edited collection "Bringing It All Back Home" (1994), Harriet Fraad and others attempt to apply the concept of class to practices in households.[7] They conclude that such an approach is certainly fruitful and explain that, from this point of view, two unequal modes of production of class exist at the same time; that, in this case, a feudal mode of production exists alongside a capitalist mode of production. This approach allows them to depict individual practices as potentially contradictory to one another, and the structures of demands placed on people who inhabit both domestic and public spaces as inhomogeneous. Their hope is that in this way, a potential for protest could emerge from the domestic sphere. This method of presentation is not incompatible with Marx, but it shifts the emphasis of the analysis from a critique of the dominant mode of rule and economy to the problem of the coexistence of different hierarchically organized relations.

Moreover, what about the accusation that Marx denied the productive character of housework and thus contributed to the devaluation of female labour? However, Marx also stated that it was bad luck, not good luck, to be a productive worker. Before I propose a different approach to the question of the function of unpaid housework for the reproduction of capitalist society as a critique of Marx, I would like to reject a number of critiques of Marx's concept of labour that have been raised in the housework debate. In my opinion, they do not refer to Marx but to the Marxism of the labour movement. That in itself would not be a problem if it were not for the fact that Marx has some important insights to offer feminists on the question of labour. So, I will proceed to reread Marx.

Let us start from the beginning. In the philosophical tradition and the more recent developments in political economy (Smith, Ricardo), Marx already found a concept of labour that was defined in contradictory ways. Labour was initially the activity of the poor; it was laborious, exhausted the spirits, or even took the place of life itself for many. However, labour was also the source of wealth and all values. Marx quotes the satirist, Mandeville:

> … but it is the interest of all rich nations that the greater part of the poor should never be idle and yet they always spend what they earn… Those who gain their lives through their daily work have nothing to motivate them to be of service except their needs, which it is prudence to alleviate, but folly would be to cure. The only thing that can make the working man hardworking is a moderate wage….From what has been developed so far, it follows that in a free nation where slaves are not permitted, the most secure wealth consists of a multitude of hardworking poor.[8]

Marx develops his concept of labour within this field of tension—labour as the link between poverty and wealth, as the contradictory basis of both. He understands labour, first and foremost, as a dimension of domination. The perspective of workers' emancipation contains general human emancipation because "the entire human bondage is involved in the worker's relationship to production and all bondage relationships are only modifications and consequences of this relationship."[9]

In his early writings, still following Hegel, Marx thinks of labour as inversion and de-realization. The inversion extends to the whole of life through an inversion of means and ends. In this context, productive participation in species life becomes a mere means of eking out life instead of realizing it.[10] This idea that labour itself is domination does not yet distinguish the material side from the economic forms and, therefore, comes to the logical conclusion that labour itself should be abolished. "It is one of the greatest misapprehensions," writes Marx in his notes on List,

> to speak of free, human, social labour, of labour without private property. 'Labour' by its very nature is unfree, unhuman, unsocial activity, determined by private property and creating private property. Hence the abolition of private property will become a reality only when it is conceived as the abolition of 'labour'.[11]

While "in all previous revolutions the mode of activity always remains unchanged and it was only a question of […] a new distribution of labour to other persons," the communist revolution "does away with *labour*."[12]

A counter-concept to (alienated) labour in the context of "universal production" is something approximating "form[ing] objects in accordance with the laws of beauty."[13] If labour is considered as capital power over people, then capital is "is man wholly lost to himself."[14]

Even in his early writings, Marx does not consider it possible to abolish labour in the sense of the productive metabolism between humans and nature; instead, by conceiving of labour as the inversion of productive activity, he compels us to reconstruct what has fallen into the form of labour and has been distorted, that is, what needs to be liberated here. In its alienated form, Marx finds: free expression of life, enjoyment of life, self-activity, participation in the human community, humanized satisfaction of needs, capacity for love,[15] all-round development of individuals, intercourse between individuals as such, conscious, free life activity as species beings.[16] The emphasis is on *free* or *self-activity*, which is conceived as species-specific. As species beings, humans are productively for each other; this determines their intercourse with one another, the community, and their development as individuals. This free activity is enjoyment. Life itself is enjoyable production.

If we start from such determinations, we can "conceive self-activity as the first need of life"; we could think of community as a productive framework; and we could also talk about the development of individuals through their own free activity—but we would never arrive at the modern sociological defence that labour should no longer be at the center of social theory (as was the case with Marx), but rather should be replaced by communication or a way of life (lifeworld). It is perfectly clear that Marx did not distinguish between the lifeworld and the world of labour, but rather sought to overthrow what is now referred to as the "lifeworld." He understands it in perspective as the enjoyable, active connection of the individuals in a community. This includes "interaction," love and life are included, although by life, Marx always means active life.

Our lives are alienated by the relations of production, by the way people produce their material lives. Simply put, throughout history, this initially meant that some indulge in free self-activity, while others produce the material existence for all.

> While in the earlier periods self-activity and the production of material life were separated since they devolved on different people, and while, on account of the narrowness of the individuals themselves, the production of material life was considered a subordinate mode of self-activity, they now diverge to such an extent that material life appears as the end, and what produces this material life, labour (which is not the only possible but, as we see, negative form of self-activity) as the means.[17]

Self-activity as a perspective of liberation related to the production of material life—this relationship is essential to even imagine a life without domination. The production of life goes through several stages—one form is that of labour. It is the most direct form of inversion, the "negative form of self-activity."[18] Thus, life is divided. In this negative form, Marx develops analytical categories that he later retains in *Capital*. The "*alienation* of the worker in his product means [...] that the life which he has conferred on the object confronts him as something hostile and alien to it," etc.[19]

Already here, we recognize his later use of language. The global condemnation of labour is replaced by the mature Marx with a differentiation between its formal determinations, on the one hand, and its natural necessity, on the other. Marx now says of labour:

> [as] useful labour, it is a necessary condition, independent of all forms of society, for the existence of the human race; it is an eternal nature imposed necessity, without which there can be no material exchanges between man and Nature, and therefore no life.[20]

Labour, therefore, always has an anthropological dimension: "By thus acting on the external world and changing it, he at the same time changes his own nature."[21]

In its alienated form, labour is two-sided. On the one hand, it produces use-values, is concretely useful, and, in this way, is independent of all social formations. On the other hand, it produces exchange values, is an expenditure of abstract human labour power, and thus forms the value of commodities. This only occurs under specific social conditions, where there is a private division of labour. The inversions or alienations arising from this context are carefully analyzed in *Capital*. The recognition of the dual character of labour is fundamental to capitalism as a commodity-producing society. However, the production of material existence as a form of free activity always remains a defining perspective for critical analysis. It contains the idea of production free of domination and, therefore, the abolition of private property (as the accumulation of exchange values) as a regulating principle, as well as the reconciliation with nature through knowledge of the laws of nature. It is a matter of bringing the purpose of the activity and the degree of expenditure into a proportion with one another, so that externally determined superordination and subordination of the tension-laden dimensions of activity are excluded. Human emancipation, therefore, lies in the developing expenditure of power for a collectively self-determined purpose. This idea connects the early and late writings.

Free life activity is understood as a process. At issue is the relationship between freedom and necessity. As one aspect of material production, the constraints of necessity should be reduced as much as possible in favor of free activity. In the realm of necessity, labour becomes a problem of distribution—everyone should perform an equal share of necessary labour. In the realm of freedom, activity is of a different kind, in which the traditional division of labour, and above all, the division between intellectual and physical labour, no longer applies. The path to this goal is through the development of productive forces that reduces the side of necessity side in the production of material life. And it also occurs through the division of human labour, its alienation. Alienated labour must be overthrown in a process in which humans ultimately appropriate the productive forces they have created. The entire relations of production must be overthrown, since these relations have perverted the human species to the point where all development, wealth, culture, and the concrete conditions of labour have been objectified against the workers and become a power over them. This contradiction can only be resolved by breaking into a new form.

In his "Critique of the Gotha Program,"[22] Marx outlines the cooperative phase of society (social ownership of the means of production), which—precisely because it emerges from capitalist society—bears the birthmarks of that society "in every respect, economically, morally, intellectually."[23] He goes on to describe a more developed "communist society," a community that has overcome the inversions of labour, and it is only in this context that we encounter the phrase about "labour as the first need of life"; "...after the enslaving subordination of individuals to the division of labour, and with it the opposition between mental and physical labour, has disappeared," labour for individuals no longer becomes "only a means of life but life's prime want."[24] These remarks have led to widespread misunderstanding. Citing Marx, individuals could be accused of being "indolent" and then "educated" to become people for whom "labour was a primary need in life." Worse still was the phrase uttered in this context: "To each according to his needs," which aroused hopes and fears that Marx might have longed for a society in which all needs formed by capitalist surplus production, and, conversely, those determined by current poverty, would be satisfied. The connection is unambiguous: if people succeed in freeing themselves from material necessity and domination through an appropriate organization of production, then the production of material life becomes a productive enjoyment and a means of developing their abilities. They will be able to live this need and, in so doing, realize their humanity. This includes the abolition of the divisions of labour, which brought about the division of human labour as the basis of social formations: the division into manual and intellectual labour, into men's and women's labour, into urban and rural labour, and finally also the hierarchical pseudo-division of labour, the class division of society into working and non-working people. With these remarks, let us turn to the questions raised previously.

It goes without saying that we cannot simply speak of labour without further ado but must always take its specific form into account—a fact that is constantly overlooked. The lack of distinction when talking about labour is the source of most misunderstandings. For example, we discuss wage labour, considering it a general determination, and use this understanding to critique the notion of labour as the primary need of life. Conversely, educating people to consider this as the primary need of life is not only pointless, but in most cases also amounts to simply teaching people to accept wage labour—an education that cannot be distinguished from submission to workplace discipline. If, on the other hand, we want to talk about the "content" that has taken the form of wage labour in our societies, I suggest using the term "self-activity in the production of material existence."

From a feminist perspective, I will now compare Marx's arguments with the feminist accusations from the housework debate. To this end, I have revisited some of his rather forgotten ideas to lend them more weight to our questions. Instead of quickly consigning Marx to the dustbin of history, I will take a step back and examine whether the women's movement could make better use of his statement about "enjoyable free activity in the production of material life." Indeed, Marx himself places the question of women's oppression in the context of alienated labour:

> This latent slavery in the family, though still very crude, is the first form of property, but even at this stage it corresponds perfectly to the definition of modern economists, who call it the power of disposing of the labour-power of others.[25]

I find it very difficult to find any basis for the accusations made by the women's movement in Marx's own statements. Although (in his early writings) he tends to favor the idea of abolishing all labour rather than simply including women's unwaged labour, there is no question that he considers a particular inversion that occurs in some human labour activities when they are converted into the form of wage labour to be the basis for the analysis of capitalist society, and not all social labour, and that this is necessary for a critique of capitalism. Moreover, is not what Marx envisioned as a future of human society and the individuals living in it constructed in such a way that the question of women's oppression, in its mixture of "natural" and social foundations, acquires an explosive dynamic? The sexual division of labour is inscribed in an almost diabolical way in the division of labour between the production of life and the production of the means of life, as well as in the further division between labour and free communal activity. The realm of real life is marginalized from the standpoint of food production and, with it, the people who primarily populate it, namely, women. At the same time, labour at the center of society is alienated, so that all hope for liberation is illusively shifted toward the living activity on the edges of society. Women, who are increasingly oppressed, are quite irrationally expected to embody the burden of society's hope for a better life, for joy, and sensual pleasure.

In Marx, we also find the formulation: "The worker therefore only feels with himself outside of his work, and in his work feels outside of himself. He feels at home when he is not working, and when he is working he does not feel at home."[26] Not without some justification, this remark also became the target of feminist critique. Does it not speak from the point of view of the male worker and overlook the situation of half of humanity who actually work at home and, therefore, work when they are at home?[27] However, such critique overlooks the problem to which Marx alludes. It is, after all, a double division: on the one hand, the separation of sensuous enjoyment and the meaning of life from labour, and on the other hand, the division of labour into paid labour and labour that is not worth anything/that counts for nothing. This is what the metaphor "he is not at home when he is working" means. In this inversion, women occupy the home, this marginal space that is also a refuge, an inverted place of hope. The oppressive idealization of women becomes essential to the survival of the male wage worker. And it is enshrined in the cooperation between the two sexes within the family. Therefore, it cannot be simply a question of naming women's labour as it occurs at home in addition to other labour, but of analyzing this contradictory tension between housework and wage work in more detail.

Would it not be revolutionary to disrupt this system as a basis for a different order? If we want to liberate the marginalized areas of life, they must be generalized and, therefore, reevaluated. At the same time, women must occupy the area of social work that is currently privileged, and its authority must also be weakened. As soon as the two sexes share the different fields of activity, an element of domination that has hitherto consolidated the old destructive order is shaken. In my view, this is a prerequisite for bringing "home back to work." This makes the women's movement crucial for the humanization of society.

The unrest that the housework debate has brought to established Marxism, despite all its problems and fruitless rejections of Marx, should be better utilized to rethink the role and function of women's oppression in the reproduction of capitalist societies. Both the early hope that Marx placed in labour and his sharp analysis of the fate of wage labour as a central source of profit and, therefore, of capitalist progress can be of current use. I do not believe that we can improve the situation of women by smuggling housework into wage labour and its laws, and thereby supplementing Marx's analysis with the problem of unpaid housework.

In my view, our critique must proceed in the opposite direction. When we attempt to understand housework itself and its role in the various stages of capitalism, we encounter an entirely different problem in Marx, which I would like to focus on below.

Family Work and Housework

We recall that the beginning of the feminist engagement with Marx was the intervention of Dalla Costa and James (1973) on the significance of the separation of the spheres of housework and factory work for the oppression of women. The ensuing debate over housework referred to Marx's analysis of wage labour. Strangely, no connection was made to his remarks on housework. I critically address this in what follows. I will begin by stating that Marx and Engels primarily use the term "housework" [*Hausarbeit*] to refer to paid work carried out in the home and treat what was usually referred to as "housework" in the 20th century as family work [*Familienarbeit*]. I will attempt to address this issue below by doubling the term "family work/housework."

In *Capital, Vol. 1*, Marx is certainly aware of family work, albeit only in passing. On the one hand, he describes the organization of labour typical of manufacturing, which took place in small family-run workshops and is still evident in agriculture today. This entailed the conversion of all time spent by family members, including children, into labour time. In connection with the enforcement of factory legislation, Marx writes:

> … when it comes to regulating the so-called 'home-labour' it is immediately viewed as a direct attack on the *patria potestas,* on parental authority. The tender-hearted English Parliament long affected to shrink from taking this step. The force of facts, however, compelled it at last to acknowledge that modern industry, in overturning the economic foundation on which was based the traditional family, and the family labour corresponding to it, had also unloosened all traditional family ties.[28]

Marx speaks here, among other things, about "the rights of children." His subject is the disintegration of the family through commodity production and, thus, the clash between two different modes of production and ways of life: the logic of the market, which presupposes the free commodity owners, and *family work* with the relative lack of rights of women and children. Elsewhere, he writes: "Previously, the workman sold his own labour power, which he disposed of nominally as a free agent. Now he sells wife and child. He has become a slave-dealer."[29] And in the footnote, he adds, "we find...traits of the operative parents in relation to the traffic in children, that are truly revolting and thoroughly like-slave dealing."[30] Marx cites a large number of factory reports, particularly on child labour, all of which show how the "the spheres of handicraft and of the domestic industries become, in a, comparatively speaking, wonderfully short time,"[31] and then comes to the well-known prospective statement:

> However terrible and disgusting the dissolution, under the capitalist system, of the old family ties may appear, nevertheless, modern industry, by assigning as it does an important part in the process of production, outside the domestic sphere, to women, to young persons, and to children of both sexes, creates a new economic foundation for a higher form of the family and of the relations between the sexes.[32]

Marx's gaze is directed forward to the organization of social production and the necessary elimination of old, hindering forms. In fact, he does not at all consider the labour done in the family apart from the production of commodities, and therefore neither how the work of caring for people and nature enters the socialization process. By *housework*, he means here paid labour within the home, the "domestic business."[33] In this context, he sometimes also speaks of "domestic industry" meaning an "outside department of the factory, the manufactory, or the warehouse."[34] Finally, two footnotes mention the area of family work outside and in conflict with wage labour outside the home. He writes about the report on the cotton crisis during the American Civil War:

> ...from a hygienic point of view, and apart from the banishment of the operatives from the factory atmosphere, the crisis had several advantages. The women now had sufficient leisure to give their infants the breast, instead of poisoning them with 'Godfrey's Cordial' (an opiate). They also had the time to learn to cook. Unfortunately, the acquisition of this art occurred at a time when they had nothing to cook. But from this we see how capital, for the purposes of its self-valorization, has usurped the family labour necessary for consumption.[35]

The conceptual proposal "family labour necessary for consumption" allows *family work* to be included in addition to wage labour, but even in this arrangement, the observation contained in the same quote that there was no "leisure" to breastfeed the infants, which is why they were "fed" in a harmful way, is overlooked. In other words, there is no starting point for the question of what actually happens to those qualities of life that are destroyed by time-savings imposed by the law of economics. Marx treats this question of breastfeeding, for example, very briefly, again as a question of wages:

> Since certain family functions, such as nursing and suckling children, cannot be entirely suppressed, the mothers confiscated by capital must try substitutes of some sort. Domestic work, such as sewing and mending, must be replaced by the purchase of ready-made articles. Hence, the diminished expenditure of labour in the house is accompanied by an increased expenditure of money. The cost of keeping the family increases, and balances the greater income.[36]

Marx's interest here lies in the fact that the inclusion of women in the process of capitalist production does not result in additional income for families and is, therefore, not really worthwhile. Nevertheless, the repeated references to substitutes leave room for further analysis.

In connection with the analysis of the division of labour, we find approaches to a theory of *family work*:

> For an example of labour in common or directly associated labour, we have no occasion to go back to that spontaneously developed form which we find on the threshold of the history of all civilised races. We have one close at hand in the patriarchal industries of a peasant family, that produces corn, cattle, yarn, linen, and clothing for home use. These different articles are, as regards the family, so many products of its labour, but as between themselves, they are not commodities. The different kinds of labour, such as tillage, cattle tending, spinning, weaving and making clothes, which result in the various products, are in themselves, and such as they are, direct social functions, because functions of the family, which, just as much as a society based on the production of commodities, possesses a spontaneously developed system of division of labour [...] The labour power of each individual, by its very nature, operates in this case merely as a definite portion of the whole labour power of the family, and therefore, the measure of the expenditure of individual labour power by its duration, appears here by its very nature as a social character of their labour.[37]

It is astonishing that Marx did not further examine this finding—that individual products are not primarily measured by the time spent on them, and therefore considered to be of greater or lesser value and compared in terms of social relevance—in terms of its consequences for the gender-specific division of labour and for the entire model of civilization. Ultimately, the calculation of time spent also turns value into a curse from which products must be protected, so that only that which consumes as little living time as possible can provide itself socially—this is the model of progress and impoverishment in one. At the same time, we also get a hint of the longing that still exists for the family today and gives it permanence as the place where production must not only be calculated in a cost-effective and labour-saving manner.

Marx does not analyze the problems that arise from the subordination of all activities not subject to the wage form to the logic of cost-benefit calculation—both in terms of the development of human beings themselves and their needs, and in terms of what is considered socially meaningful and recognizable. His enthusiasm for comprehensive economization essentially subordinates all labour and its evaluation to the concept of rationalization, which he considers necessary in order to satisfy further "life demands":

> The more the productiveness of labour increases, the more can the working day be shortened; and the more the working day is shortened, the more can the intensity of labour increase. From a social point of view, the productiveness increases in the same ratio as the economy of labour, which, in its turn, includes not only economy of the means of production, but also the avoidance of all useless labour.[38]

In his detailed analyses of labour under capitalism, the gender-specific division of labour is only mentioned in passing. He describes its emergence as initially a "natural[]" division "based on a purely physiological foundation," that develops into mutually interdependent branches through exchange.[39] He does not further examine the arrangement of these areas, which is central to the capitalist model of civilization. The fact that Marx did not pursue his reflections on the dominant character of the gender-specific division of labour (see above), as outlined in particular in the *German Ideology*, is all the more striking given that this formed the basis for the development of a social formation in which society essentially produces that generates profit, so that all work that cannot follow this temporal logic, that cannot be rationalized, cannot be automated or accelerated—such as caring and nurturing people and nature—is left lying, destroyed, or left to the unpaid care of women. Today, we can probably assume that the crises of uncontrolled and unfettered development of productive forces and the overexploitation of nature and its resources are connected to this logic and order of spheres, to which the oppression of women owes its origin. In this respect, we can conclude, sharpening our critique of Marx, that a one-sided analysis of wage labour instead of the connection between socially necessary labour and its superordination and subordination leads to an inadequate analysis of the reproduction of capitalist societies, and thus of their duration and the forces that support them. From a feminist perspective, therefore, there is much to be reworked and restructured here.

In Marxism, there are no further analyses of the relationship between family work and wage labour—studies of *women's work* in the family became the special domain of ethnologists.[40] Rosa Luxemburg follows Marx's view on this point, seeing the family as something from which women have already been "torn."[41] Lenin, too, is only interested in the family as a place of dullness from which women could be rescued.

It was only in the 1980s that women's studies began to consider linking the form of *family work* with an analysis of social conditions. Maria Mies,[42] Veronika Bennholdt-Thomsen,[43] Claudia von Werlhof,[44] and others suggested that a generalization of subsistence work could provide a solution to the global problem that developed from commodity production and progressed to the exploitation of the Third World. Unfortunately, this proposal to return to a stage before commodity production does not contain any indication of how to proceed and how the world population can be fed on this basis.

Looking back at the development of humanity from today's perspective, we see that only those activities and associated needs that could survive in the market (i.e., that were worthwhile in terms of time spent) developed. All production and activities whose specific nature required an extensive expenditure of time without a correspondingly large product fell by the wayside. It is logical that the majority of agricultural activities, as well as forestry and care for nature, and even raising children, are incompatible with the logic of time reduction.[45] To the extent that the products obtained in this way are indispensable for human survival, even in the short term, this development drives a division of humanity into those who can prove themselves on the market and those "sub-humans" who labour below the level of average people. This heralds the advent of "third worlds" and their impoverishment. In first-world countries, development is more complicated. On the one hand, women have a hard time supporting themselves when they have to engage in "unremunerative activities"; this is true even if they have an "additional" job. A husband economically cushions her position, who appears, as already in Marx and Engels, as the breadwinner of the family. However, a large part of these, let us call them "time-consuming" activities, remain undone. Thus, the development of humanity goes hand in hand with its brutalization. Entire continents are exposed to starvation, and in developed capitalist countries, entire generations of young people are denied entry into society. Instead, there is an increase in narcotics and drugs and corresponding crime. The signs that the capitalist civilization model, in which human development is subordinated to an extremely rationalized expenditure of labour time and the products and needs that can only be produced in this way, which are driving us into war, crisis, and barbarism, are becoming increasingly evident during times of crisis. The progress of the material productive forces does not free people to take their development as human beings into their own hands. They lack the time. Thus, it remains a by-product of general industrial development and women's labour. In this context, it also seems logical that Gorbachev, for example, hoped to remedy the neglect of young people by encouraging women to return to their families. In this way, Fourier's statement that the degree of human development can be inferred from the degree of women's emancipation remains highly relevant. It concerns the relationships between people, their needs, their relationship to their sensuality, to the nature around them, to the work of their hands and heads, and even to themselves as human individuals.

Notes

1 Editors' Note: The text was first published as "Feministisch Arbeiten mit Marx," in *Utopie Kreativ*, no. 109/110 (1999), 125–137. It has also been republished in *Der im Gehen erkundete Weg: Marxismus–Feminismus* (Argument Verlag, 2015), 308–324.

The original German text opens with a poem by Volker Braun, who is a German prize-winning poet, playwright, and novelist currently residing in Berlin. His writings explore themes of fate, immovability and acceptance as part of the political question. During the 1980s he worked closely with German philosopher, Wolfgang Fritz Haug.

What did he take from us?
of effort, this spongy Hercules
But what did he leave to us? What lack of illusions.
What a global loss
On safe values. Which spread
Inability to submit!
And how impossible, between us
Not to doubt everything. Since then
All our successes: only advance payments
Of history. Then the time
Not giving in to the matter
And how impossible not to go to the end: and it not for him
beginning to hold

[Was hat er uns abgenommen
an Mühe dieser schwammige Herkules
Aber was hat er uns überlassen. Welchen Mangel an Illusionen.
Welchen weltweiten Verlust
An sicheren Werten. Welch verbreitete
Unfähigkeit, sich zu unterwerfen!
Und wie ausgeschlossen, unter uns
Nicht an allem zu zweifeln. Seither
All unsere Erfolge: nur Abschlagszahlungen.
Der Geschichte. Dahin die Zeit
Sich nicht hinzugeben an die Sache
Und wie unmöglich, nicht ans Ende zu gehen: und es nicht für den
Anfang zu halten].

2 See Frigga Haug, *Frauen-Politiken* (Argument, 1996).

3 Mariarosa Dalla Costa, "Women and the Subversion of the Community," *The Power of Women and the Subversion of the Community*, ed. Selma James (Falling Wall Press, 1973), 21–56. Translator's Note: Mariarosa Dalla Costa is an Italian feminist and co-founder of the 1972 International Feminist Collective based in Padua. The focus of the collective was to generate debate and discussion regarding housework which gave emergence to the International Wages for Housework initiative and campaign.

4 Claudia von Werlhof, "Der blinde Fleck in der Kritik der politischen Ökonomie," *Beiträge zur feministischen Theorie und Praxis*, no. 1 (1978): 18–32.

5 Sigrid Pohl, *Entwicklung und Ursachen der Frauenlohndiskriminierung. Ein feministisch-marxistischer Erklärungsansatz* (Lang, 1984).

6 This appropriation of protests formerly intended to liberate women, continues. However, in March 1999, the representative of the Austrian right-wing party in Kärnten, Jörg Haider, won 42% of the vote by, among other things, promising to pay for housework. In 2012, the government bloc brought the childcare allowance to the German Bundestag, which also set out to pay for part of the housework.

7 Harriet Fraad, Richard Wolff and Stephen Resnick, *Brining It All Back Home: Class, Gender & Power in the Modern Household* (Pluto Press, 1994).
8 Bernard de Mandeville, *The Fable of the Bees* (London, 1728), 212, 328, quoted in Karl Marx, *Das Kapital, Marx Engels Werke Band 23* (Dietz, 1962), 643; Karl Marx, *Capital Volume 1, Marx and Engels Collected Works: Volume 35* (International Publishers, 1976), 610.
9 Marx, Karl "Ökonomisch-philosophische Manuskripte," *Marx Engels Werke Band 40* (Dietz, 1968), 467–588, 521; Karl Marx, "Economic and Philosophic Manuscripts of 1844," *Marx and Engels Collected Works, Volume 3: Karl Marx March 1843-August 1844* (International Publishers, 1976), 229–346, 283.
10 Marx, "Manuskripte," 516; Marx, "Economic and Philosophic Manuscripts of 1844," 276.
11 Karl Marx, "Über F. Lists Buch 'Das nationale System der politischen Ökonomie'," *Beiträge zur Geschichte der Arbeiterbewegung*, Heft 3/1972, 14. Jg. (Dietz, 1845): 425–446; Karl Marx, "Draft of an Article on Friedrich List's Book: Das Nationale System der Politischen Oekonomie," *Marx and Engels Collected Works, Volume 4: Marx and Engels 1844–45* (International Publishers, 1976), 265–293, 278.
12 Karl Marx, "Die Deutsche Ideologie," *Marx Engels Werke Band 3* (Dietz, 1969), 9–439, 69; Karl Marx, "The German Ideology," *Marx and Engels Collected Works, Volume 5: Marx and Engels 1845–47* (International Publishers, 1976), 23–439, 52.
13 Marx, "Manuskripte," 517; Marx, "Economic and Philosophic Manuscripts of 1844," 277.
14 Marx, "Manuskripte," 523; Marx, "Economic and Philosophic Manuscripts of 1844," 283.
15 Karl Marx, "Auszüge aus Mills 'Éléments d'économie politique'," *Marx Engels Werke Band 40*, 445–463, 462; Karl Marx, "Comments on James Mill 'Élémens d'économie politique'," 211–228, 228.
16 Marx, "Manuskripte," 516; Marx, "Economic and Philosophic Manuscripts of 1844," 276.
17 Marx, "Die Deutsche Ideologie," 67; Marx, "The German Ideology," 87.
18 Marx, "Die Deutsche Ideologie," 67; Marx, "The German Ideology," 87.
19 Marx, "Manuskripte," 511; Marx, "Economic and Philosophical Manuscripts of 1844," 272.
20 Marx, *Das Kapital,* 57; Marx, *Capital,* 53.
21 Marx, *Das Kapital,* 57, 192; Marx, *Capital*, 187.
22 See Karl Marx, "Kritik des Gothaer Programms," *Marx Engels Werke Band 19* (Dietz, 1962); Karl Marx, "Critique of the Gotha Program," *Marx and Engels Collected Works, Volume 24: Marx and Engels 1874–83* (International Publishers, 1976).
23 Marx, "Kritik des Gothaer Programms," 20; Marx, "Critique of the Gotha Program," 85.
24 Marx, "Kritik des Gothaer Programms," 21; Marx, "Critique of the Gotha Program," 87.
25 Karl Marx, "Die Deutsche Ideologie," 32; Marx, "The German Ideology," 46.
26 Marx, "Manuskripte," 514; Marx, "Economic and Philosophic Manuscripts of 1844," 274.
27 See Rada Ivekovic, "Noch einmal zum Marxismus und Feminismus," *Geschlechterverhältnisse und Frauenpolitik,* Argument-Sonderband 110 (Argument, 1984): 103–112.
28 Marx, *Das Kapital,* 513; Marx, *Capital*, 491.
29 Marx, *Das Kapital*, 418; Marx, *Capital*, 399.
30 Marx, *Das Kapital*, 418; Marx, *Capital*, 399.
31 Marx, *Das Kapital*, 514; Marx, *Capital*, 493.
32 Marx, *Das Kapital*, 514; Marx, *Capital*, 492.
33 See Marx, *Das Kapital*, 316, 363f, 489–493, 533, 629, 699, 733, 776; Marx, *Capital*, 448, 348f., 468–472, 511, 598, 662, 697, 720.

34 Marx, *Das Kapital*, 485. See also 533, where he is interested in housework as a "hybrid form"; it is not directly subordinate to capital, but rather "usurers" or "merchants" guarantee the pressure on domestic producers; Marx, *Capital*, 463, 511.
35 See Marx, *Das Kapital*, 416; Marx, *Capital*, 397.
36 See Marx, *Das Kapital*, 417; Marx, *Capital*, 399.
37 Marx, *Das Kapital*, 92; Marx, *Capital*, 399.
38 Marx, *Das Kapital*, 552; Marx, *Capital*, 530.
39 Marx, *Das Kapital*, 372; Marx, *Capital*, 356.
40 See Claude Meillassoux, *Die wilden Früchte der Frau*. Über häusliche Produktion und kapitalistische Wirtschaft (Syndikat, 1983).
41 Rosa Luxemburg, "Die Proletarierin," *Gesammelte Werke Band 3: 3. Juli 1911 bis Juli 1914* (Dietz, 2002), 410; Rosa Luxemburg, "The Proletarian Woman," *The Rosa Luxemburg Reader*, ed. Peter Hudis and Kevin B. Anderson (Monthly Review Press, 2004), 243.
42 Translator's Note: Maria Miles (1931–2023) was a German professor of sociology, a Marxist ecofeminist, an activist for women's rights, and an author. She spent quite a lot of time in India which inspired her to write about Indian women's experiences of labour, unionisation, and lack of security.
43 Translator's Note: Veronika Bennholdt-Thomsen is an ethnologist and sociologist committed to the German women's studies movement. Much of her work focuses on rural women's experiences.
44 Translator's Note: Claudia von Werlhof is a German sociologist and political scientist. Together with Maria Mies and Veronika Bennholdt-Thomsen, she is a co-founder of the ecofeminism movement. Specifically, her work intersects the Third world, women's experiences, and ecological questions.
45 Some attempts to industrialize agriculture have produced those horrible products that Brecht curtly predicted: "You will no longer recognise the fruit by its taste." See Bertolt Brecht, *Schriften zur Literatur und Kunst, Band 1: 1920–1939* (Aufbau-Verlag, 1966), 185.

References

Brecht, Bertolt. *Schriften zur Literatur und Kunst, Band 1: 1920–1939*. Aufbau-Verlag, 1966.

Dalla Costa, Mariarosa. "Women and the Subversion of the Community." In *The Power of Women and the Subversion of the Community*. Edited by Selma James. Falling Wall Press, 1973.

De Mandeville, Bernard. *The Fable of the Bees: or, Private Vices, Publick Benefits*. J. Tonson, 1728.

Fraad, Harriet, Richard Wolff, and Stephen Resnick. *Bringing It All Back Home: Class, Gender & Power in the Modern Household*. Pluto Press, 1994.

Haug, Frigga. *Frauen-Politiken*. Argument, 1996.

Haug, Frigga. "Feministisch Arbeiten mit Marx." *Utopie Kreativ*, no. 109/110 (1999): 125–137.

Haug, Frigga. *Der im Gehen erkundete Weg: Marxismus–Feminismus*. Argument Verlag, 2015.

Ivekovic, Rada. "Noch einmal zum Marxismus und Feminismus." In *Geschlechterverhältnisse und Frauenpolitik*, Argument-Sonderband, no. 110 (1984): 103–112.

Luxemburg, Rosa. "Die Proletarierin." In *Gesammelte Werke*, Band 3: 3. Juli 1911 bis Juli 1914. Edited by Annelies Laschitza and Günter Radczun. Dietz, 2002.

Luxemburg, Rosa. "The Proletarian Woman." In *The Rosa Luxemburg Reader*. Edited by Peter Hudis and Kevin B. Anderson. Monthly Review Press, 2004.

Marx, Karl. *Das Kapital. Marx Engels Werke, Band 23*. Dietz, 1962a.

Marx, Karl. "Kritik des Gothaer Programms." In *Marx Engels Werke, Band 19*. Dietz, 1962b.

Marx, Karl. "Auszüge aus Mills 'Éléments d'économie politique.'" In *Marx Engels Werke, Band 40*. Dietz, 1968a.

Marx, Karl. "Ökonomisch-philosophische Manuskripte." In *Marx Engels Werke, Band 40*. Dietz, 1968b.

Marx, Karl. "Die deutsche Ideologie." In *Marx Engels Werke, Band 3*. Dietz, 1969.

Marx, Karl. "Über F. Lists Buch 'Das nationale System der politischen Ökonomie.'" *Beiträge zur Geschichte der Arbeiterbewegung*, Heft 3/1972, 14. Jg. (1972): 425–446.

Marx, Karl. *Capital Volume 1, Marx and Engels Collected Works: Volume 35*. International Publishers, 1976a.

Marx, Karl. "Comments on James Mill, Éléments d'économie politique." In *Marx and Engels Collected Works, Volume 3*. International Publishers, 1976b.

Marx, Karl. "Critique of the Gotha Program." In *Marx and Engels Collected Works, Volume 24: Marx and Engels 1874–83*. International Publishers, 1976c.

Marx, Karl. "Draft of an Article on Friedrich List's Book: Das Nationale System der Politischen Oekonomie." In *Marx and Engels Collected Works, Volume 4: Marx and Engels 1844–45*. International Publishers, 1976d.

Marx, Karl. "Economic and Philosophic Manuscripts of 1844." In *Marx and Engels Collected Works, Volume 3: Karl Marx March 1843–August 1844*. International Publishers, 1976e.

Marx, Karl. "The German Ideology." In *Marx and Engels Collected Works, Volume 5: Marx and Engels 1845–47*. International Publishers, 1976f.

Meillassoux, Claude. *Die wilden Früchte der Frau. Über häusliche Produktion und kapitalistische Wirtschaft*. Syndikat, 1983.

Pohl, Sigrid. *Entwicklung und Ursachen der Frauenlohndiskriminierung. Ein feministisch-marxistischer Erklärungsansatz*. Lang, 1984.

Von Werlhof, Claudia. "Der blinde Fleck in der Kritik der politischen Ökonomie." *Beiträge zur feministischen Theorie und Praxis*, no. 1 (1978): 18–32.

Chapter 10

Engels' Problem with the Woman Question[1]

Frigga Haug

Preliminary Remarks

I joined the socialist wing of the student movement at the end of the 1950s, which was then known as the SDS (Socialist Democratic Student Union). The women's movement only began at the end of the 1960s. Although I was involved from the very beginning—after all, the women's movement initially developed from the left-wing student movement—this autobiographical precursor to socialist thinking determined my first steps in the cause of women's liberation. Consequently, like most women's groups at the time, I began to find support for women's emancipation in the socialist classics: Bebel and Engels in particular. My memories of both are highly ambivalent. Still ignorant about almost all issues that concerned me as a woman, I was thrilled to find entire books on "the woman question" and felt noticed and at home. On the other hand, I also remember how terribly tedious and laborious I found reading Engels' *Origin of the Family*. We studied the book in a working group. And as if it were yesterday, I can still feel the effort of wading through the Iroquois gens,[2] the Punaluan family,[3] and the uncle-aunt sibling marriages, to finally arrive at questions that concerned us. It was like an obstacle course toward a goal whose illuminating and liberating quality we somehow never achieved. I pushed the experience with the book aside. Later memories were fleeting, and I dismissed them as a failure on my part to be interested in ethnological studies. But a thorn remained.

This year, on the 100th anniversary of Engels' death, I felt I owed it to myself and to Engels to reexamine what this original text contained. I wonder whether Engels, as a theorist of women's liberation, had provided us with unfulfilled potential and tools worth considering, treasures that we failed to uncover at the time, or whether he obscured women's liberation thinking in the labour movement through the specificity of his approach. I am aware that this question is somewhat ahistorical. After all, we live in different times and different realities, which make it crystal clear that women's oppression is at the heart of the formation of society and its functioning, whereas in Engels' time, liberation thinking had only just begun to explore the horizons of capital and labour. Nonetheless...

DOI: 10.4324/9781003480143-10

Gender Relations and Labour

I studied *The Origin of the Family* once again in 1995 and arrived at rather strange experiences and results, which I would like to formulate below as preliminary theses.

While the Iroquoian gens, the Punaluan family and the like did not bore me in the slightest, nor was their presentation arduous and laborious, I stumbled, right at the beginning, over the formulation of the problem as outlined by Engels. The foreword states:

> The less labour is developed and the more limited the volume of its products and, therefore, the wealth of society, the more predominantly the social order appears to be dominated by ties of kinship. However, within this structure of society based on ties of kinship, the productivity of labour develops more and more; with it, private property and exchange, differences in wealth, the possibility of utilising the labour power of others, and thereby the basis of class antagonisms: new social elements, which strive in the course of generations to adapt the old structure of society to the new conditions, until, finally, incompatibility of the two leads to a complete transformation. The old society, based on ties of kinship, bursts asunder with the collision of the newly developed social classes; in its place a new society appears, constituted in a state, the lower units of which are no longer groups based on ties of kinship but territorial groups, a society in which the family system is entirely dominated by the property system, and in which the class antagonisms and class struggle, which make up the content of all hitherto written history now freely unfold.[4]

Although at first glance this seems to be a good research guide, upon closer inspection, one recognizes a line of thought that Engels largely follows, which inevitably led to a blind spot—the overlooking of the oppression of women. In short, Engels offers an explanation here that suggests that social regulation occurred through ties of kinship [*Geschlechtsbande*], kinship relationships [*Verwandschaftsverhältnisse*], and families up until the point when labour took over the regulation of class relations. Such a framework leads to forgetting an analysis of labour in societies where kinship relationships, ties of kinship, prevail, and, conversely, to foregoing an analysis of "ties of kinship" in societies where labour, property, and class are conceived as determining. In the following, I will show that this is precisely the case in Engels's work and, to a large extent, in that of his successors, where the woman question is almost systematically excluded from most dimensions. There is an additional, almost linguistic, peculiarity. Engels uses the term gender relations [*Geschlechterverhältnisse*] to refer to the question of the reproduction of the species and the relations associated with it, which I still find valid today and even consider a key term.[5] In the context of ancient societies, which are supposed to be regulated by kinship relationship [*Verwandtschaftsbeziehungen*], he speaks of ties of kinship and kinship associations. Strangely, these terms slip into one another in such a way that, at the moment when he speaks historically of the dominance of labour in the regulatory context, the disappearance of the analysis of kinship associations also means that gender relations largely disappear. According to the logic of the research outline, gender relations can hardly have any social relevance with the advent of value-producing labour.

In the same preface, this point is reinforced by how Engels takes up and develops the arguments of "The German Ideology" concerning the reproduction and production of life. He outlines what is meant by "production and reproduction of immediate life"[6]: "On the one hand, the production of the means of subsistence, of food, clothing and shelter and the implements required for this; on the other, the production of human beings themselves, the propagation of the species."[7] He refers to both as "productions" and, in doing so, provides a starting point for a theory of women's oppression—one whose elaboration he himself, however, obstructs by subsequently defining the two types of production, in their further development, as "the development of labour, on the one hand, and of the family, on the other."[8] By making such a distinction between labour (which is concerned with food, clothing, housing, etc.) and family, he leaves the latter, and consequently the theory of women's oppression, with nothing but the organization of biological processes and their legalization and nationalization. *Family labour* cannot be thought. Consequently, in the *Origins*, he examines the organizations of reproduction, but not the relation between labour performed within the family and the overall labour and the reproduction of society.

This is made easier by the fact that the concepts of *production of life*, *creation of human beings*, and the *reproduction of the species* are kept at such a level of generality that the entire process and the domination and oppression, labour and exploitation embedded in it are swallowed up.

Engels works alongside the common thinking of Marxism about social relations and dominant regulations and, within them, forms that are advanced in such relations. He thus assumes that "the productivity of labour" develops in a society structured on the basis of kinship ties, and with it, "private property and exchange, differences in wealth, the possibility of utilizing the labour power of others, and thereby the basis of class antagonisms."[9] Here, he develops a network of determinations that are familiar to us today as central to Marxist analysis and social reality, but which he then conceives of as all being emancipated from ties of kinship—so gender relations no longer appear. They are replaced by the state and classes. This arrangement makes it almost impossible to think of the state as permeated by gender relations, that is, as a patriarchal state; and it took nearly 100 years before attempts were made to cautiously extend the concept of class or class struggle to gender struggles, and thus to place the latter in a systemic context of capitalism.[10] This, incidentally, is despite the fact that Engels himself notes at least a simultaneous occurrence of women's oppression and class antagonism: "The first class antithesis which appears in history coincides with the development of the antagonism between man and woman in monogamian marriage, and the first class oppression with that of the female sex by the male."[11] However, this observation has little impact on his further presentation and analysis of the shift in the regulation of society. The very idea of assuming a shift in dominance in the regulation of society and, at the same time, a change, a different linking of previously existing practices and classifications, still seems to me fruitful. Only, for Engels, this goes hand in hand with showing little or no interest in labour relations determined by these bonds in a society based on "ties of kinship," and, conversely, no interest in the continued effect of gender relations in a society based on labour. In the "complete revolution" he thus loses sight of important determining factors.

Elsewhere, however, in connection with the further development of society, Engels was quite clear that labour also takes place within the family. Looking back historically, he says in *Anti-Dühring* that

> The whole development of human society beyond the stage of brute savagery begins on the day when the labour of the family created more products than were necessary for its maintenance, on the day when a portion of labour could be devoted to the production no longer of the mere means of subsistence, but of means of production.[12]

However, Engels is not interested in the significance of this process for the remaining part, which he calls the "production...of the mere means of subsistence," but focuses solely on social progress, which comes from the surplus of the product of labour over the maintenance costs of labour, as the basis of all "social, political and intellectual progress."[13]

It is interesting to look closely at how he describes labouring for subsistence, that is, the procurement of necessary food and clothing, and where the transition to surplus production, property, and wealth begins:

> Now, with herds of horses, camels, donkeys, oxen, sheep, goats and pigs, the advancing pastoral peoples...acquired possessions demanding merely supervision and most elementary care in order to propagate in ever-increasing numbers and to yield the richest nutriment in milk and meat....Hunting, once a necessity, now became a luxury.[14]

The thrust is clear. In the shift in the source of food from the daily repetition of hunting to the self-reproducing basis of domestic animals, Engels wants to outline a revolution which led to a new social order based on property. But he does so with words that distract from labour and, simultaneously, from the question of gender relations in this labour. To put it bluntly, one could say that this paves the way for the neglect of housework in favor of the analysis of the overall social labour and the prospect of liberation. In the brief mention of supervision and the most elementary care, one can still imagine elements of labour, even if these immediately appear diminutive; the remaining part of the necessary labour, the preparation of food until it can be eaten, disappears entirely as a subjective act. The animals deliver themselves, almost as in a fairytale. Among other things, milking, cleaning out the stables, herding the cattle, slaughtering and skinning, and the actual preparation of food also disappear. In short, the labour assigned to women disappears, as if its products were simply natural wealth.

On the other hand, hunting appears as a genderless luxury, as if those who have gradually become wealthy could take part in it in their spare time, regardless of their gender and position in the whole.

Engels states that new property dominates the family order and that the new owners are the male heads of the family because "[a]ccording to the division of labour then prevailing in the family," they were responsible for procuring food and women for household goods.[15] The subjugation of the female sex finds a vague and almost fairytale-like explanation at this point. The sexes [*Geschlechter*] appear as two brothers, one of whom suddenly finds gold in his field, while the second only stones and therefore does well to submit to the former if he wants to share in the wealth and survive. Without being able to elaborate this point here, this unconditional assignment of food procurement to men seems historically just as unlikely as the tasks in the home are underdetermined by the implicit statement that they do not bring wealth. Overall, the formulation of the problem is geared toward excluding activities that are not carried out in the form of paid labour from the analysis of the overall social production process, thereby considering them as negligible for the functioning of the whole.

The question of the interaction between patriarchy and capital is obscured. And the ground is prepared for the illusion that a family without property, that is, the proletarian family, would be free of domination.

Today, we can assume that the domination/subjugation relations were also expanded in the proletarian family to the detriment of women. With advancing industrialization, growing prosperity even among the working class, and the possibility of living on just one income, that of the man, the position of the proletarian housewife also increasingly deteriorated. Engels does indeed mention the male breadwinner's wage and the "domestic slavery of women," but he does not consider these phenomena as sufficient to provide his analysis with a theoretical framework that allows for the development of the proletariat while maintaining patriarchy.[16]

In a society where care and being cared for are neither provided for nor even contradict the dominant regulations, one must expect that the privilege of being cared for will be seized upon. The analysis should therefore show the shift from regulation based on to ties of kinship to labour based on property, and thus determined by property, primarily as a shift in the goals of social action. The determining factor is no longer the question of the reproduction of the species but rather the accumulation of wealth. This makes it all the more important to include in the analysis the fate of activities that do not create wealth, such as caring for the next generation, and their relationship to labour that is recognized as dominant. This separation-connection is central to the definition of patriarchal capitalism, yet it remains largely relegated to a blind spot in Engels' arrangement of the problem.

With the replacement of the dynamics of kinship associations by those of property, and thus of class struggles, we arrive, as Engels writes, to the "content of all hitherto *written* history."[17] This formulation already reveals a correction to Marx and Engels' earlier view that all history is the history of class struggles. In any case, this shift was not sufficient to counteract the arrogance with which the labour movement relegated all questions of gender relations to prehistory, thereby deeming them irrelevant to real political questions.

Another line of thought in Engels concerns the development of productive forces.[18] The focus is on the specifics of the product and production rather than on the arrangement in which this occurs. It remains to be seen whether this history will be written not only as a positive history of human development but also as a specific history of inequality and underdevelopment.[19]

The *Origin* also contains a grandiose and frequently quoted formulation of the "*world-historic defeat of the female sex*"[20] through the overthrow of mother right. The next sentence follows: "The man seized the reins in the house too, the woman was degraded, enthralled, became the slave of the man's lust, a mere instrument for breeding children."[21] The spontaneous sympathy with the women's solidarity expressed in the sentence conceals the fact that there is no talk of struggles, weapons, or perpetrators (except in the mode of seizing). Women appear in the familiar position…as victims.

There are other lines of argumentation in this text that are not simply wrong, but that point toward a problematic direction in theoretical work and politics. For example, when men's wage labour is paralleled with the prostitution of women, right up to the idea that women are selling their morals, not their labour power:

> In both cases, this marriage of convenience often enough turns into the crassest prostitution—sometimes on both sides, but much more usually on the part of the wife, who differs from the ordinary courtesan only in that she does not hire out her body, like a wage worker, on piecework, but sells it into slavery once and for all.[22]

As much as we may agree with the statements about loveless, property-based marriage as prostitution, it is nevertheless true that in this perspective, unpaid labour, that part of the total social labour that is the condition for the concentration on the efficiency, rationalization, and, consequently, the reduction of wage labour, disappears amidst the moral outrage.

There is a far-sighted definition of the problematic relation between public and private that hints at the political significance of housework, which is precarious and yet to be grasped theoretically. Engels writes:

> In the old communistic household, which embraced numerous couples and their children, the administration of the household, entrusted to the women, was just as much a public, a socially necessary industry as the procurement of food by

> the men. This situation changed with the patriarchal family, and even more with the monogamian individual family. The administration of the household lost its public character. It was no longer the concern of society. It became a *private service*. The wife became the first domestic servant, pushed out of participation in social production.[23]

Nevertheless, nothing more follows from this outline of the problem. As is well known, Engels' analysis culminates in the vision of a fully industrialized society, which later served as the model for the Soviet Union. The abolition of housework as a prerequisite for the emancipation of the female sex was the motto that, to my knowledge, was only questioned by Gorbachev, far too late and, again, in a distorted form.[24]

In Engels appears the oft-quoted sentence as a prescient formulation:

> The emancipation of women becomes possible only when women are enabled to take part in production on a large, social scale, and when domestic duties require their attention only to a minor degree. And this has become possible only as a result of modern large-scale industry, which not only permits of the participation of women in production in large numbers, but actually calls for it and, moreover, strives more and more to reduce private domestic duties to a public industry.[25]

I consider this to be a mistake which also establishes a politics that is altogether questionable because it disregards the position and function of women's unpaid labour in the capitalist mode of production.

Capitalist production requires the constant incorporation, exploitation, and colonization of non-capitalist modes of production. I have argued elsewhere[26] that a profit-oriented economy based on reducing living labour and growth poses a problem for carrying out the time-consuming maintenance and care work necessary for survival. One solution is to hand over a portion of these tasks to women, who are thereby unable to act as equal and free wage workers; another part is wrested from the welfare state as a form of compromise, part is exported to the Third World, and a part remains undone, a corrosive element of modern societies. Even in these brief remarks, it should be clear that this arrangement itself constitutes domination, produces a particular form of exploitation, is prone to crises, and, at the same time, is the very scene of crises, as is evident today.

Notes

1 This text was published in German as "Problematik der Frauenfrage," *Zwischen Utopie und Kritik. Friedrich Engels—ein 'Klassiker' nach 100 Jahren*, ed. Theodor Bergmann, Mario Keßler, Joost Kircz, and Gert Schäfer (VSA-Verlag, 1996), 42–50.

2 Translator's Note: In Iroquois society, a 'gens' (also known as a clan) is a collective of people who trace their descent through the female matriarchal line, sharing a common

name and obligated to mutual support and protection, especially in avenging perceived or real injuries.

3 Translator's Note: In pre-missionary Hawaiian culture, 'punalua' refers to a group marriage where multiple brothers are married to multiple sisters, or where husbands and wives are from different kinship groups, with the two or more husbands of a wife, or the two or more wives of a husband, being considered 'punalua' to each other.

4 Friedrich Engels, "Der Ursprung der Familie, des Privateigentums und des Staats," *Marx Engels Werke, Band 21* (Dietz, 1962), 28; Frederick Engels, "The Origin of the Family, Private Property and the State," *Marx and Engels Collected Works, Volume 26: Engels 1882–89* (International Publishers, 1976), 132.

5 Editors' Note: While English differentiates between 'sex' and 'gender,' the German word *Geschlecht* can refer to both. In "The Origin of the Family" Engels uses the term *Geschlechtsbande* (often translated in English as kinship ties or ties of kinship), *Geschlechterverbänden* (translated in English as either, once again, kinship ties, or as kinship groups or kinship associations), and *Geschlechtsverhältnisse* (typically translated in English as sexual relations). However, he does not use the term *Geschlechterverhältnisse*, which is typically rendered in English as gender relations. In keeping with previous translations of Frigga Haug's work, in which the term *Geschlechterverhältnisse* is rendered as "gender relations," this translation also renders all references to *Geschlechterverhältnisse* as "gender relations."

6 Engels, "Der Ursprung der Familie," 27; Engels, "The Origin of the Family," 131.

7 Engels, "Der Ursprung der Familie," 28; Engels, "The Origin of the Family," 131.

8 Engels, "Der Ursprung der Familie," 28; Engels, "The Origin of the Family," 132.

9 Engels, "Der Ursprung der Familie," 28; Engels, "The Origin of the Family," 132.

10 See Jacques Kergoat, "Luttes de classe: quelques problems," *L'Homme et la société*, no. 117–118 (1995): 57–64.

11 Engels, "Der Ursprung der Familie," 68; Engels, "The Origin of the Family," 173.

12 Friedrich Engels, "Anti-Dühring," *Marx Engels Werke, Band 20* (Dietz, 1975), 1–303, 180; Friedrich Engels, "Anti-Dühring," *Marx and Engels Collected Works, Volume 25: Engels* (International Publishers, 1976), 1–309, 180.

13 Engels, "Anti-Dühring," *Marx Engels Werke*; Engels, "Anti-Dühring," *Marx and Engels Collected Works*.

14 Engels, "Der Ursprung der Familie," 58; Engels, "The Origin of the Family," 162.

15 Engels, "Der Ursprung der Familie," 59; Engels, "The Origin of the Family," 164.

16 Engels, "Der Ursprung der Familie," 75; Engels, "The Origin of the Family," 181. In contrast to this position see Dorothy Smith, "The Deep Structure of Gender Antitheses: Another View of Capitalism and Patriarchy," *Humanity & Society* 8, no. 4 (1984): 395–402.

17 Engels, "Der Ursprung der Familie," 28; Engels, "The Origin of the Family," 132.

18 Engels, "Der Ursprung der Familie," 33; Engels, "The Origin of the Family," 136.

19 The *Origin* also contains a number of interesting and expandable theoretical proposals, which I will not go into in detail in this context. For example, Engels understands kinship as a system, family as a dynamic form–a problem arrangement that helps to decipher otherwise incomprehensible relationships of non-simultaneity and at the same time allows a direction of development to be identified.

20 Engels, "Der Ursprung der Familie," 61; Engels, "The Origin of the Family," 165.

21 Engels, "Der Ursprung der Familie," 61; Engels, "The Origin of the Family," 165.

22 Engels, "Der Ursprung der Familie," 73; Engels, "The Origin of the Family," 179.

23 Engels, "Der Ursprung der Familie," 75; Engels, "The Origin of the Family," 179.

24 Gorbachev had proposed to enable women to better fulfill "their everyday duties at home—housework, the upbringing of children and the creation of a good family atmosphere." He wanted to solve problems: "in children's and young people's behavior, in our

morals, culture and in production [...]-partially caused by the weakening of family ties and slack attitude to family responsibilities." Mikhail Gorbachev, "Mikhail Gorbachev on Women and the Family," *Population and Development Review* 13, no. 4 (1987): 757–759, 758. For this he needed women and their indispensable educational function as mothers and housewives. See Frigga Haug and Barbara Ketelhut, "Die Perestrojka und die Frauen," *Das Argument* 30, no. 4 (1988): 507–512.

25 Engels, "Der Ursprung der Familie," 28; Engels, "Origin of the Family," 262.

26 Haug, "Ökonomie der Zeit, darin löst sich alle Ökonomie auf. Neue Herausforderungen an einen sozialistischen Feminismus," *Das Argument* 184, no. 6 (1990): 879–894.

References

Engels, Friedrich. *Der Ursprung der Familie, des Privateigentums und des Staats. Marx Engels Werke, Band 21.* Dietz, 1962.

Engels, Friedrich. *Anti-Dühring. Marx-Engels-Werke, Band 20.* Dietz, 1975.

Engels, Friedrich. *The Origin of the Family, Private Property and the State. Marx and Engels Collected Works, Vol. 26: Engels 1882–89.* International Publishers, 1976a.

Engels, Friedrich. *Marx and Engels Collected Works, Volume 25: Engels.* International Publishers, 1976b.

Gorbachev, Mikhail. "Mikhail Gorbachev on Women and the Family." *Population and Development Review* 13, no. 4 (1987): 757–759.

Haug, Frigga. "Problematik der Frauenfrage." In *Zwischen Utopie und Kritik. Friedrich Engels–ein 'Klassiker' nach 100 Jahren.* Edited by Werner Bergmann, Mario Keßler, Jan Willem Kircz, and Lothar Schäfer, 42–50. VSA-Verlag, 1996.

Haug, Frigga, and Barbara Ketelhut. "Die Perestrojka und die Frauen." *Das Argument* 30, no. 4 (1988): 507–512.

Haug, Frigga, and Barbara Ketelhut. "Ökonomie der Zeit, darin löst sich alle Ökonomie auf. Neue Herausforderungen an einen sozialistischen Feminismus." *Das Argument* 184, no. 6 (1990): 879–894.

Kergoat, Jaques. "Luttes de classe: quelques problèmes." *L'Homme et la société*, no. 117–118 (1995): 57–64.

Smith, Dorothy. "The Deep Structure of Gender Antitheses: Another View of Capitalism and Patriarchy." *Humanity & Society* 8, no. 4 (1984): 395–402.

Chapter 11

The Neoliberal Project

The Male Concept of Work and the Overdue Renewal of the Gender Contract[1]

Frigga Haug

Work and Hope

One of the problems in the discussion about the future of work is the unspoken charge of the concept of work. It is often accompanied by the word full employment, a term that is full of hopes, experiences, and aversions. Full employment is "never achievable anymore," as the media and politicians claim, and the actual developments show it very clearly, so everyone must realize that hope for this situation is illusory. The farewell comes with mixed feelings because the word also resonates with what no one can want. Being employed, busy around the clock, being fully occupied, sounds like therapy, like being cared for, like a distraction, or at least like being controlled by others. Why should everyone be fully employed? The answer seems simple at first: of course, because of the need to secure one's existence. Being employed, being occupied, means having a job that pays, pays one's bills, and more. Conversely, if someone is not fully employed, they may not be perceived as competent and cannot fully count on social recognition. In this view, work is also linked to social protection.

However, at the same time, almost everyone today knows or feels and believes that work is something strenuous, a serious contrast to fun play, which one should avoid as long as possible. Work is the opposite of leisure, vacation, and extended happiness, so why not make the most of a situation where society appears to be running out of work, at least work for everyone, and stop looking for work?

In this emotionally difficult situation, in which work is not only a self-evident right of members of society but is also associated with a range of negative feelings, it is difficult to progressively discuss the threat posed by the slogan of *the end of the working society* with positive passion or righteous indignation. The right to work or work for all are easier to dismiss with derision in the mass media as productivism, the destruction of nature, and the consumption of resources than to be constructively linked to the transformation of society.

My first hypothesis is that the reality of a range of wage labour jobs and the discourse around work have created a climate in which important positions that are indispensable for the renewal of the working society have already been lost and abandoned.

DOI: 10.4324/9781003480143-11

Distrust of work is acquired individually and is a product of the experience of actual work activities and their embeddedness in a social context. It is, therefore, instructive to take a step back and remember. I will briefly describe such a step back.

We—me and a group of students in a second-chance education seminar—set ourselves the task of writing down our memories of encounters with the concept of work. The result was astonishing in every way. To summarize very broadly: all childhood memories of work were positive, associated with expansion, happiness, belonging, freedom, growing up, togetherness, being loved, becoming independent, and skills. In terms of **form**, as could be expected with children, work was by no means tied to wages, and in terms of **content**, it was all more desirable the more new things could be learned from it, the more it was done together with others, the more useful and therefore meaningful it was for everyone. Of course, this does not remain the case; in all work biographies, a change occurred long before work took the form of wage labour, but certainly by then. It is easy to calculate that all the above-mentioned determinations of content and form are or must be gradually relinquished over the course of life, and that this is sufficient to instill an attitude and view that largely associates work with negative connotations. In this way, one can understand in detail that the negatively connoted forms and contents of work are themselves a critique of specific kinds of work and not a mere rejection of it.

I formulate my second thesis: We can assume that the desire to work as well as its avoidance, or shirking, are cut from the same cloth. A blind dialectic develops within the structures of social life. Suddenly and unexpectedly, enthusiasm for work turns into its opposite. The practical solution of seeking real life outside of work comes up against limits everywhere, as well as willing but unwanted concessions, such as those encapsulated in the term unemployment.

In addition to remembering ourselves, conceiving ourselves as historical figures with a semi-conscious knowledge of the material from which we made ourselves, we can go back to the infancy of critical theory. It is helpful to re-read what Marx thought and wrote about social problems. In the field of labour in particular, he is known as someone who linked labour together with self-realization but also with alienation; someone who could not conceive of life without labour precisely because human beings, as natural beings, must earn their living through labour. Today, it is common practice to throw Marx onto the rubbish heap of history; in terms of work, he lands there softly upon the one-third or half of humanity that has already been discarded or is slated for discard, for whom no work is supposedly available. The throwaway movement is accompanied by an echo of hope, of being freed from work and finding liberation beyond it, and, indeed, the necessity of doing so.

Before we rashly agree with this, let us briefly clarify what Marx actually thought about work and what we throw away when we free ourselves from the tiresome context of work. He emphasized the importance of understanding work in the specific form in which it is carried out, for example as wage labour, as slave labour, as labour imposed by others, and of examining the inversions that arise as a result of the determinacy of the form in individual moments of labour, and thus from which the shackles of human activity would therefore have to be freed. For him, the alienated form of labour contains: free expression of life, enjoyment of life, the activity of the human community, self-activity awareness of having satisfied a human need, knowing oneself to be confirmed in love[2]; the development of individuals into total individuals; the intercourse of individuals as such[3]; conscious, free life activity as a species being,[4] and much more. The emphasis is on "free activity" or "self-activity"—this is always conceived of in relation to the species and as a species-specific characteristic. As species beings, humans are productively active for each other; this determines their intercourse, the community, and the development of individuals. This self-activity is enjoyment. Life itself is a pleasurable production. The organs of human individuality are seeing, hearing, smelling, tasting, feeling, thinking, observing, experiencing, wanting, acting, and loving.[5]

These Marxist definitions are entirely compatible with the childhood memories of work mentioned above. From these two "sources," I formulate a third thesis: work and enjoyment have become separated. Bringing them back together remains a prospect for liberation. This project is incompatible with settling into a society in which some engage in wage labour and others profit from it, some are only provided for, and still others toil from morning to night without having wage labour and without really being provided for.

This is another peculiarity in the discussion of the future of work and the corresponding society. Despite more than 20 years of feminist discussion—which in turn only reiterated what has been an unmistakable reality since the beginning of industrialization, i.e. since the ever-solidifying separation of production and reproduction—despite the undeniable existence of unpaid female labour in our society, which is dominated by wage labour (regardless of whether we call it housework, reproductive labour, or family work), the discussion, thinking, and action about work in society and its decline remains almost exclusively about paid wage labour. The development here has been strangely schizophrenic. After about 20 years of debate on housework, the notion that women lie on the couch at home and eat chocolates can no longer be propagated so cheaply. Everyone is now ready to recognize housework as work in principle; housewifery is seen as a profession that no longer has to be mentioned with embarrassment, and there are increasing reports about the economic value of women's unpaid work in the home. According to UNPD calculations, this amounted to 11,000 billion dollars worldwide in 1995. This amount of work and money is invisible in the debate about the future of the working society, which accounts for a good half of the total social product.[6] However, even though such calculations are already official government numbers, even though the media themselves speak of unpaid housework in terms of recognition, even though, unlike 20 years ago, there is no longer any significant resistance to mentioning housework, the public economic and political discourse on work remains entirely unaffected by this. When discussing the future of societal work, the focus is always and inevitably on paid wage labour, usually in the form of so-called full-time work. The underlying concept of work is purged of all caring, reproductive, and responsible activities for oneself, for one's offspring, and for the rest of nature, with which one must also engage in a caring, "sustainable" way for one's own life. In short, the concept of work in this form presupposes the delegation of caring activities to other non-workers. In this way, we can certainly say that it is a male concept of work, an access to an expenditure of labour power that can only sustain itself on the basis of unnamed women's work outside the wage labour cycle.

By disregarding at least half of all socially necessary activities, a plausible calculation of the structural necessity of increasing unemployment is presented. Political discourse is structured in such a way that we are suddenly forced to look at a company's balance sheet, without, of course, being asked whether the product created there is meaningful, useful, or pointless and harmful. We are supposed to worry about sales and profit margins and, above all, to find both wage costs and non-wage costs too high and, therefore, to participate in the calculation that this company cannot afford its workers in the long term. Three hundred thousand are to be laid off, or only 18,000—we have long since become accustomed to incredible numbers and are forced to imagine a society in which, to continue operating in the same way, and better and more productively, at least a third of its members must be weeded out as superfluous parasites. Once we have accepted this level of calculation, it becomes difficult to think of and implement alternatives if we do not consider the stoker on the electric locomotive from the Second Industrial Revolution to be a possible solution.

I cautiously formulate a fourth hypothetical question: Can we actually afford companies that operate according to profit and productivity/growth standards while practicing this economic model as social politics? Can we afford politics that prepares for such deregulation and privatization? This raises the question: What about the second half of the work activities mentioned above, which are socially necessary but unpaid? Or, more simply, what benefit does the reduction of work to the male concept of work have for the functioning of current industrial societies?

The Neoliberal Project

I turn to the authorities concerned with the question of future planning. That is, I study the neoliberal project as it is currently sweeping across the globe. In their recently published book on globalization, Altvater and Mahnkopf provide a comprehensive scenario based on a large amount of facts and figures.[7] Despite a chapter on women's employment relations, this useful book does not fundamentally address the question of socially necessary total labour and the role of women in it. I will therefore revisit the neoliberal project in a microanalysis. I present the draft of the neoliberal economic wing in a small country, Switzerland, to illustrate and facilitate discussion of "world trends" in this context.

I am referring to the small volume with the telling title *Courage to Depart*, edited by leading economists and business leaders in Switzerland, and to discussions in this context.[8] To get straight to the point: the book is not a particularly strong example of neoliberal rhetoric, but it certainly carries the current buzzwords on its flag—or rather, on its cover: economic liberalization, a quantum leap in information technology, globalization, liberalization, democracy, motivation, and entrepreneurial initiative. The goals are also familiar: companies need more attractive location conditions, then the economy will grow, prosperity for all, and employment.

Such slogans remain persistent and seem logically compelling, even if they can easily be refuted as counterfactual. For example, the average return on capital has not decreased since 1970, yet there is no boom. It is now also common knowledge that increasing productivity with a growing return on capital does not necessarily create jobs. Conversely, "prosperity for all" is the euphemistic term for a development with an ever-widening gap between the wealthy and an ever-growing proportion of the poor. We also already know from experience that the combination of government cutbacks and the unleashing of market forces create ever more unemployment and more and more unfinished work.

As a Swiss product, free from the abrasions and controversies of the European Union, this "regulatory" draft is initially more "open," more straightforward, and more ruthless.

First, as with the concept of work in politics, I will attempt to discuss the question of consent. I ask myself what is convincing and appealing about the neoliberal model. Therefore, I examine the concept in terms of populism and hegemony.

When Margaret Thatcher was still relatively new to government, one of the populist arguments she used to win the hearts of her audience, even though she was announcing unpopular cuts to the national budget, was that running a state was just like managing a household. You simply cannot spend money you have not earned.[9] This makes sense to everyone, as it brings the dimensions of politics and the larger economy into the realm of common sense that is accessible to everyone. Apart from the fact that this is not true, as a certain amount of national debt is one of the characteristics of healthy economies, the argument creates proximity and understanding, bringing politics into the everyday realm of possibility. (Incidentally, our media, which is repeatedly providing us with new examples of why it is imperative for companies to lay off employees, proceeds in a very similar way.) How does the Swiss White Paper operate at this level?[10]

The widening gap between global politics and everyday local life is unceremoniously bridged, and the global heaven of wealth, growth, competition, and the market is to be reached by invoking the virtues of each individual. The stance taken on the side of individuals is both understandable and therefore populist, and it poses a threat to those who are unwilling or unable to comply.

If we look at the appeals to Switzerland as a nation, we learn about the entrepreneurial spirit, self-confidence, openness and innovation, a change in mentality and course corrections—all expressed dynamically in soccer terms; for example, avoiding sliding into midfield, taking the lead—and looming danger is painted if Switzerland does not keep up with international competition: a billion working-age people from Latin America and Asia are pushing their way onto the global economic markets. After introducing some well-known information about information technology, the book finally states: "This paves the way to a global, uniform marketplace that is simultaneously open to everyone."[11]

Such equality and opportunity speak for individuals and their virtues as follows: a departure from vested interests, courage, personal responsibility, freedom of choice, mature citizens who themselves contribute to solving the problem of the lack of lifelong jobs, e.g. not being a burden to anyone, joining forces with close ones for mutual support, and not delegating anything to politics; being willing to perform, not wanting to be anonymous, experiencing humanity and, if they are socially disadvantaged, seeking personal attention. Otherwise, individuals have the opportunity to teleshop and balance their work, family, and leisure time by working on a networked home monitor.[12] The whole thing is called personal lifestyle.

These invocations are somewhat vague, predominantly moral, and overly general, but they are the only point at which individuals are even considered as members of society in the "regulatory model" [*ordnungspolitischer Entwurf*].

The increasing globalization of the economy and politics also means an increase in distance and thus detachment from one's existence in everyday local life, which, in concrete terms, experiences whatever happens to it as fate. In a draft that aims to make the politics of capital and the state's response to it understandable to the masses, it is therefore useful to study how this bridge from the global economy to the lives of individuals is built. In the Swiss context, it works like this: insofar as globalization appears both as a reality and an opportunity, it is about expanding markets, location issues, competing, and offering high-quality products. The highest degree of distrust is appropriate here because all these terms are worn-out platitudes placed over a sea of crimes, or at best twists and distortions, behind which other human dramas are playing out. There are several proposals, even demands, to deal with the issue of foreigners—still referred to here as foreign workers—in a different, more liberal way. This refers, on the one hand, to what is known as brain drain, the recruitment of highly qualified workers from abroad, and, on the other hand, to the weakening of unions as collective bargaining partners. A free market for wage labour.

Market expansion—e.g., Latin American and Asian markets are enticing—growth and prosperity are everywhere. Does anyone who has witnessed the growing misery of Mexico, the model student of neoliberal politics, still believe this? What is beginning to emerge here is a gruesomely mirrored there: the wealth of one group is bought at the price of the mass misery of about half the population.

Location and competition. The terms sound solid in a sporty way. The advantage of location to emerge victorious in competition seems to be planned in the same way as the hedgehog dealt with the hare. As expected, location is linked to non-wage labour costs and the state's "unnecessary social expenditures." Here, then, the members of society finally reappear, as those who work and those who consume undeservedly, who are a burden.

The necessary conclusions are easy for anyone to draw: from the standpoint of a functioning economy in the microelectronic age, which wants to emerge as a constant winner on the world market and thus grow and make further profits, the members of society must be divided into two groups: those who are highly qualified and highly motivated to continue learning and researching using all technical means and to launch new products onto the market, faster, better, and higher—physical fitness is complemented by that of the brain and character. And those who take responsibility for their miserable situation into their own hands, supported by the care of others like them and who don't expect anything more than to die discreetly.

Therefore, in many places in the White Paper, the state is called upon to discontinue payments in various sectors because they are considered bureaucratic, anonymous, and counterproductive insofar as they fail to encourage a willingness to perform on the part of those who have fallen by the wayside. The proposals largely correspond to the practices already initiated by the conservative parties, including those in coalition governments in Europe and Germany.

A study of global employment relations shows that the real winners are the highly skilled workers. Needless to say, they are predominantly white and male. Where women's work exists to a relevant extent and increases periodically, it is entirely unskilled work or work that is not considered to require any qualification, such as childcare and elderly care. Employment is correspondingly precarious. The employee structure is laying off its midfield, leaving behind their Olympic team and maintenance assistants. I will come back to what this means for women. First, let us look at how the Swiss manifesto deals with this development. There is indeed one aspect of the proposals that is appealing in the short term—the question of qualifications. Where the productive forces are deduced from the mode of production of the microelectronic age and considered from the standpoint of labour that is needed to be carried out on them it is, on the one hand, simply a matter of importing labour—i.e., brain drain—and, on the other hand, it places demands on the school and university system, which sound like they are worth supporting. In the future, the focus should be on learning *how to learn* rather than on specific subjects that quickly become outdated. Borders should be made permeable, comprehensive job profiles developed, research strengthened, and there should be less state involvement in universities—in other words, autonomy? The catch is that all training is to be linked to the economy, privatized, and subject to performance criteria. At first glance, this has three immediate consequences, among a variety of effects that need to be discussed on a larger scale.

1 This type of qualifying training does not apply to everyone; instead, it exacerbates the division of humanity into those who succeed and those who are ultimately left behind. To illustrate this, imagine that in a country like Mexico, where the use of microelectronics is naturally at the highest level, and where the internet has become more prevalent at universities than in prosperous Germany, yet at the same time, about half of the population can neither read nor write (meaning that the productive forces have not made the transition from the level of agrarian to industrial society and are probably also not intended to do that).

2 Connecting everything to the economy reduces, is one-sided, atrophies human abilities, and hinders human development—I am referring to the development of skills and activities in art, music, literature, movement, thinking, philosophy, shaping society, etc., all of which are economically superfluous.
3 Applying performance criteria to learning processes is counterproductive. Speed, output, and rationalization make creativity impossible, which requires leisure, a change in learning efforts, and dreams. Even those who succeed in the privatized economy linked to performance institutions miss the goal of being human by a wide margin. Learning urgently needs to be freed from the competitive and profit-driven private sector.

The Swiss draft is intended as a project for the future. I would therefore like to remind you of the questions about the concept of work, which still await answers, as well as about women's unpaid labour and its future.

The assessment for the project of humanity or a human future is extraordinarily meagre. It is the only point in the book at which people of the next generation are mentioned. Cast aside are those called upon to take responsibility for themselves, those without jobs. Women remain almost entirely unmentioned. We did not expect that a text written so exclusively from the standpoint of a few high-tech companies to address gender relations or attribute an important role to the female population in its regulatory ideas—but not a single positive mention, and no space to locate them at all?

At second glance, however, women or "femininity" appear everywhere as an invisible background, as a basis, when it comes to providing caring assistance for socially marginalized men, so that these men do not anonymously and parasitically fatten themselves under the state's watering can principle.[13] One suspects that the state's social dismantling will not only come at the expense of women but is also expected to be made socially tolerable by them.

Difficulties in caring for the elderly and securing pensions in the event of illness make it worthwhile to take a look at the human possibility of working without pay or wage claims. It is supposed to sound charitable that not everything has to be regulated materially. And what if the majority of women are ending up unemployed anyway?

The suspected stopgap role assigned to women, who after all make up half of the population in Switzerland, sheds a stark light on the planned economic and social model. The only thing that should count is what pays off for those who benefit from it. The only guiding principle is profit-orientation in growth sectors—everything else is left behind. The unfinished work in the home, reproduction, social affairs, and nature conservation is assigned to the rest of the discarded population in the name of responsibility, not even love. Even the emissions tax is to be abolished. And the future, in whose name this is to be done, is being abolished. In the effort to subjugate the remnants of the state to the conditions and needs of the growth industries, the word is given to further dehumanization, destruction, and annihilation of humanity. The need for a political-ethical solution, which is becoming increasingly urgent at every turn and due to the globalization of capital, information, and technical possibilities, is to be obscured by the timely dismantling of the state. This is the project.

American writer Marge Piercy has transformed such a horror vision, as outlined in the "regulatory model," into a futuristic novel of frightening reality. *He, She, and It* is set in 2056, the Earth is in a state it will end up in if we continue as we are, if neoliberal practices prevail.[14] Nuclear power plants and hidden bombs have gone off somewhere—most of the earth is uninhabitable, devastated, polluted, and diseased. A good two-thirds of the surviving humanity vegetate there, partly mutated, adapted to the terrible conditions of crime, disease, and horribly ravaged nature. What remains are a few global capitals (such as Siemens and Toshiba) that do what they have always done in their sealed cities and on satellites: they produce and make profits. This is achieved at the highest level of the development of productive forces with correspondingly highly qualified workers, all of whom have undergone numerous mechanical modifications and are kept fit. The differences between robots and humans are fluid—a human project, a meaning nowhere noticeable except for a tiny ghetto of Jews, also in an artificial world, and a resistance emerging from the sea of horrors on earth called "Glop." Against this backdrop, in this scenario, not only does the realistic nature of such a development become apparent, but also, above all, that this future must be stopped, that we must discuss how we want and can live, what the standards of societies and the economy must be. And, of course, that we cannot, under any circumstances, leave this to the growth aspirations of capital.

Instead, the lives of future generations must be just as much a guiding principle for our creative endeavors as a meaningful task for ourselves, who are the present generation. Therefore, it is no coincidence that women in the *Courage to Depart* are explicitly only included where they "impair the competitiveness of the Swiss economy": in the demands to lift the ban on night work, abolish maternity insurance, and raise women's retirement age. This makes it possible to exclude all questions about people's lives today and tomorrow.

Proclaiming the global as immediate without mediating it with the local disempowers local people and makes their lives appear as fate. Capital production as the only regulating principle of society, known as the free market economy in the high-tech age, automatically relegates a large portion of the population to the rubbish heap. Among them are the women who, at best, remain eligible for free, marginal repairs. However, hardly anyone can place their hope on lifelong breadwinners anymore, as lifelong jobs no longer exist even for men. Omitted in the Swiss Awakening as representative of the neoliberal project are: the woman question, social and ecological problems, and the Third World—in other words, all the burning questions.

As a highly brief thesis from this discussion, I would formulate the following: the neoliberal project is a social plan that seeks to replace social humanity with an autonomous economy of growth, competition, and profit as the supreme regulatory authority for global society. Any alternative proposal must question neoliberalism as a whole.

Politics around a New Gender Contract

In this context, it seems essential to address the question of gender relations as a foundation of neoliberal economics, a shackle that hinders alternative thinking and action. Not only the male concept of work and the associated resistance to a different structure of the working society but also a brief examination of the neoliberal project pointed to the increasing exclusion and neglect of essential areas of life for which women are ultimately made responsible. When the genders begin to examine their relations, the relations of society as a whole once again come into focus as something that urgently needs to be challenged. This sentence contains hopes that need to be explained:

1 That the dynamics of gender relations make new beginnings and changes at least conceivable for society as a whole;
2 That from the standpoint of both genders, changes in production and gender relations are desirable;
3 That rebellion in the socio-political landscape is conceivable at all. The fact that this should or could be discussed politically under the gender contract necessitates a preliminary remark about today's struggles for and within contractual thinking.

At this point, I do not intend to offer a lesson on contractual thinking and the various discussions about the social contract, but assume this is largely known. Criticism and general distrust also seem justified, but the social battlefields have shifted to such an extent that even the individual issues that seemed hardly worth fighting over can now be used differently as critique and for emancipatory purposes. In this way, I follow Altvater and Mahnkopf in their assessment that the current mobilization for the construction of a new social contract from left to right is simultaneously a position of resistance against the tendencies of economic globalization.[15] Whether we are talking about the *Alliance for Work* or the *North-South Treaty*, the ecological-social *New Deal,* or the social-ecological generational contract, it is always somehow a matter of defending the common good against the dominance of special interests. In neoliberal thinking, a social contract cannot be articulated; this is the moral deficit of the neoliberal construct.

If the struggle over the social contract already harbors dimensions of civil resistance, despite its conservative overtones, this is all the more true when such movements are strengthened by including the problem of gender relations and simultaneously subversively undermined. First, it is undeniable that the genders are in a contractual state that is partly practically fixed and partly secured at least culturally. It is essentially based on a kind of division of labour for different responsibilities and duties in society and can be updated in the current upheavals as well as serves as an outlet and supposed solution for socially produced incompatibilities. On the one hand, it seems that the so-called housewife marriage in Western Europe has given way to more dynamic models of women's claims to paid jobs and their own lives, at least since the 1970s. On the other hand, these shifts seem to have remained entirely superficial, as the consensus is that the ever-increasing unemployment should be endured without any significant protest at the expense of women. The term dual earner is being used again, corresponding to the rejection of jobs for women who already have a husband with a job. It is not just the resistance to quotas for women in politics, business, and science that stubbornly persists; but conversely, the fight for them is weakened by the general cultural consensus that we currently have more important, more existential problems. And in the government-backed deregulation measures favoring capital locations, which we also know under the collective slogan of dismantling the welfare state, it is, as shown above, tacitly assumed that the (unemployed) women will find themselves stepping in to help in places of misery that have been torn open: be it in child care, caring for young people, the elderly, the disabled, the sick, the unemployed, the mentally disturbed, and so on. Against all odds, there remains hope and consensus that women could and should assume such responsibility for living beings. To the extent that they agree to this without significant resistance, they contribute to maintaining the current practice of subordinating society to the economic objectives of a few as a possible social project in which people could live.

Under a new gender contract,[16] the social project would have to be discussed again. I do not imagine that contracts based primarily on the division of labour would be concluded and that the relations between the genders would be subject to new regulations; rather, gender relations, which leave social organization to the pursuit of growth and profit in a way that is both blocking and unbearable, will be called up anew. First and foremost, it must be about making a contract with the future and turning the question of the next generation, the reproduction of the species, and the problem of how and under what conditions the next generation should grow up, into a political question. It is of utmost importance for civil society what the coming generation will be like since it is not only the distant future but also the already present. The responsibility for future generations cannot be left to women on the basis of a private division of labour since they cannot bear such responsibility. Ultimately, this encompasses questions concerning education, nutrition, the environment, resources, urban development, and so on. We can narrow down the problem to all political and economic questions that are today regulated according to criteria that are largely incompatible with the future of humanity. Terminating an existing gender contract in which women are absurdly responsible for the future without having the slightest competence and power does not mean that they too should be integrated into the paid workforce on equal footing, while free work, voluntary work, and unfinished work remain undone. After us, the deluge. Instead, it means actually taking on these responsibilities and gaining the corresponding power and authority to do so. It is about a different division of power and work, which must negotiate a different social model, set different priorities, and position the genders differently. It seems essential that the male gender takes part in such a changed objective. This would only be the beginning of a human society.

In public discussions, which could be held anywhere, political learning processes would have to be carried out, and concrete and realistic individual demands would have to be made from comprehensive plans for a society worth living in. These could already be parts of a larger contract, such as the women's quota, qualification opportunities, and even tax policy, without the entirety of such a gender contract having to retain the cold dimensions of exchange and the market. The contract form serves here to actually include everyone involved as self-confident political actors and, in contrast to the feelings that it connotes, is not intended to elevate the realm of the political and personal into the economic world of detached, soulless actions, but rather to bring it down into the discussion of the members of society.

The starting point would be an understanding of the totality of necessary social work, which would include caring for future generations and, therefore, also caring for the environment as a prerequisite for the survival of future generations. It would certainly be a different political society with different priorities that holds up a mirror to the current one with an inventive and socially critical intention.

The concept of the contract would thus be useful in several ways. From a social perspective, it is a utopian vision and a warning for today's politics. If we radicalize and intensify the current problem areas by fundamentally including gender relations, a society emerges on the horizon that differs fundamentally from today's society, especially in terms of its objectives and thus also in terms of everyday domination. The essential regulatory instruments would no longer be profit and growth but rather questions about the quality of our present and future lives and species reproduction, that is, questions about the future. How time is used is essential, whereby the question of usefulness loses its purely utilitarian content and becomes a question of the quality of life. The division of labour becomes a question of justice and diversity. It becomes nonsensical to restrict the concept of work to wage labour without requiring all work to be paid. The possibility of not being able to exist independently in a society where everyone works would be unthinkable. Once a political goal, the quota becomes a self-evident prerequisite for a society that is a project of its members and thus loses its rigid, dogmatic character. Society as a utopian project can also be further imagined by women. There are plenty of models for this.[17] In current realpolitik, the concept of the contract is once again becoming a compromise form of direct intervention. This, in fact, includes quotas for women in all jobs and, conversely, quotas for men in the reproductive and social spheres. This would include the right to work and to politics for both genders.

Since, according to all previous analyses, we must assume that the genders have opposing viewpoints and positions in society and that these gender relations are intertwined with relations of production, the genders are collective actors who would have to regulate the new social contract consensually. In doing so, both genders have something to lose and something to gain so that society as a whole can survive. Such contract negotiations, struggles, and planning would essentially be a new and different politicization of the public sphere. This is not primarily a tug-of-war between the actors. It is about bringing the current crisis points into the public discussion so that the participation of the evolved constellations—here, that of the genders—in the untenable conditions becomes obvious, as does their potential to participate in change. The premise is that we actually live in a patriarchal capitalism that has ultimately marginalized even survival as a private matter. This needs to be turned on its head.

Notes

1 Editors' Note: This text is based on a presentation given by Frigga Haug at the Lake Constance Conference of the German Green Party on the September 29, 1996.

2 Karl Marx, "Auszüge aus Mills, *Éléments d'économie politique,*" *Marx Engels Werke Band* 40, *Supplementary Volume I* (Dietz Verlag, 1968), 462; Karl Marx, "Comments on James Mill, *Élémens d'économie politique,*" *Marx and Engels Collected Works, Vol. 3: Karl Marx March 1843-August 1844* (International Publishers, 1975), 228.

3 Karl Marx, "Deutsche Ideologie," *Marx Engels Werke Band 3* (Dietz Verlag Berlin, 1978), 68; Karl Marx, "The German Ideology," *Marx and Engels Collected Works, Vol. 5: Marx and Engels 1845–47* (International Publishers, 1976), 88.

4 Karl Marx, "Ökonomisch-philosophische Manuskripte," *Marx Engels Werke Band 40,* 516; Karl Marx, "Economic and Philosophic Manuscripts of 1844," *Marx and Engels Collected Works, Volume 3* (International Publishers, 1976), 275.

5 Marx, "Ökonomisch-philosophische Manuskripte," 539; Marx, "Economic and Philosophic Manuscripts of 1844," 299–300.

6 United Nations Development Program, *Human Development Report 1995* (Oxford University Press, 1995).

7 Elmar Altvater and Birgit Mahnkopf, *Grenzen der Globalisierung* (Westfälisches Dampfboot, 1996), 58.

8 David de Pury, Heinz Hauser und Beat Schmid (eds.), *Mut zum Aufbruch: eine wirtschaftspolitische Agenda für die Schweiz* (Orell Füssli, 1995).

9 For this, see Stuart Hall, *The Hard Road to Renewal: Thatcherism and the Crisis of the Left* (Verso Books, 1988).

10 Editors' Note: The so called Swiss *White Paper [Weißbuch]* refers to the *Courage to Move Forward* [*Mut zum Aufbruch*] book, published in December 1995 and edited by David de Pury, Heinz Hauser, and Beat Schmid. The book outlines an economic policy agenda for Switzerland, which was signed by sixteen other prominent figures from business and academia and sparked widespread and controversial debate.

11 De Pury, Hauser and Schmid, *Mut zum Aufbruch, 20.*

12 De Pury, Hauser and Schmid, *Mut zum Aufbruch*, 51.

13 Editors' Note: The German expression *watering can principle [Gießkannenprinzip]* describes a method of allocating grants or subsidies in which neither the order of applications nor the urgency of the individual cases plays a decisive role. The key feature of this approach is that funds are spread evenly across all recipients—figuratively "poured out like from a watering can"—without assessing actual needs or distinguishing between more and less urgent situations.

14 Marge Piercy, *Er, Sie und Es* (Argument, 1993).

15 Elmar Altvater and Birgit Mahnkopf, *Grenzen der Globalisierung*, 58.

16 See on this also Janna Thompson, "Wollen Frauen den Gesellschaftsvertrag neu fassen?," *Das Argument,* no. 210 (1995): 497–512.

17 Marge Piercy, *City of Darkness, City of Light* (Fawcett Columbine, 1996); Ursula K. Le Guin, *The Left Hand of Darkness* (Orbit, 1981).

References

Altvater, Elmar, and Birgit Mahnkopf. *Grenzen der Globalisierung. Ökonomie, Ökologie und Politik in der Weltgesellschaft.* Westfälisches Dampfboot, 1996.

de Pury, David, Heinz Hauser, and Beat Schmid, eds. *Mut zum Aufbruch: Eine wirtschaftspolitische Agenda für die Schweiz.* Orell Füssli, 1995.

Deutsche Gesellschaft für die Vereinten Nationen. "Bericht über die menschliche Entwicklung 1995." UNO-Verlag, 1995.

Deutsche Gesellschaft für die Vereinten Nationen. *United Nations Development Program.* "Human Development Report 1995." Oxford University Press, 1995.

Hall, Stuart. "Der Thatcherismus und die Theoretiker." In *Ausgewählte Schriften. Ideologie, Kultur, Medien, Neue Rechte, Rassismus.* Edited by Nora Räthzel. Argument Verlag, 1989.

Haug, Frigga. "In der Arbeit zuhause sein?" In *Erinnerungsarbeit.* Argument, 1990.

Haug, Frigga. Stichwort Arbeit." In *Kritisches Wörterbuch des Marxismus, Band 1.* Edited by Wolfgang Fritz Haug. Argument, 1996a.

Haug, Frigga. "Politik um einen neuen Geschlechtervertrag." In *Frauen-Politiken.* Argument, 1996b.

Le Guin, Ursula. *Planet der Habenichtse.* Heyne, 1981.

Piercy, Marge. *Er, Sie und Es.* Argument, 1993.

Piercy, Marge. *Frau am Abgrund der Zeit.* Argument, 1996.

Marx, Karl. "Auszüge aus Mills, *Éléments d'économie politique.*" In *Marx Engels Werke Band 40.* Dietz Verlag, 1968a.

Marx, Karl. "Ökonomisch-philosophische Manuskripte." In *Marx Engels Werke, Band 40.* Dietz Verlag, 1968b.

Marx, Karl. "Comments on James Mill, *Éléments d'économie politique.*" In *Marx and Engels Collected Works, Volume 3.* International Publishers, 1975a.

Marx, Karl. "Economic and Philosophic Manuscripts of 1844." In *Marx and Engels Collected Works, Volume 3: Karl Marx March 1843–August 1844.* International Publishers, 1975b.

Marx, Karl, and Friedrich Engels. "The German Ideology." In *Marx and Engels Collected Works, Volume 5: Marx and Engels 1845–47.* International Publishers, 1976.

Marx, Karl, and Friedrich Engels. "Die deutsche Ideologie." In *Marx Engels Werke, Band 3.* Dietz Verlag, 1978.

Thompson, Janna. "Wollen Frauen den Gesellschaftsvertrag neu fassen?" *Das Argument,* no. 210 (1995): 497–512.

Chapter 12

From the Fisherman and His Wife[1]

Frigga Haug

The Fisherman and His Wife[2]

Once upon a time there was a fisherman who lived with his wife in a piss pot near the sea. Every day the fisherman went out to fish, and all he did was fish and fish. One day he was sitting with his line and gazing into the clear water. And all he did was sit and sit. Suddenly his line sank deep down to the bottom, and when he pulled it up, he had a large flounder on the line, and the flounder said to him, "Listen here, fisherman, I beg of you, let me live. I'm not a real flounder but an enchanted prince. So what good would it do you to kill me? I certainly wouldn't taste very good. Put me back into the water, and let me go."

"Hold on," said the man. "You don't have to waste your words on me. I would have thrown a talking fish back into the water anyway."

He then put the fish back into the clear water, and the flounder swam to the bottom, leaving behind a long streak of blood. Then the fisherman stood up and returned to the piss pot to be with his wife and told her that he had caught a flounder but since it had been an enchanted prince, he had let him go.

"Didn't you wish for anything?" asked the wife.

"No," said the husband. "What should I have wished for?"

"Ah," said the wife. "Don't you think it's awful that we've got to live in this piss pot? It stinks, and it's disgusting. You should have wished for a little hut. Go back and call him. Tell him we want a little hut. I'm sure he'll give us one."

The husband didn't think that this was the right thing to do, but he went back to the sea anyway, and when he arrived, the sea was green and yellow, and he stood on the shore and said:

"Flounder, flounder, in the sea,
if you're a man, then speak to me.
Though I don't agree with my wife's request,
I've come to ask it nonetheless."

The flounder came swimming up to him and said, "Well, what does she want?"

DOI: 10.4324/9781003480143-12

"Oh," said the man, "my wife, Isabel, thinks I should have wished for something because I caught you. Since she doesn't want to live in a piss pot, she'd like to have a hut."

"Just go home," said the flounder. "She's already got it."

The fisherman went home, and his wife was standing in the doorway of a hut and said to him: "Come inside, husband. Look! Now, isn't this much better?"

There was a stove and a parlor, also a kitchen. Behind the hut was a little yard and garden with all kinds of vegetables and chickens and ducks.

"Oh," said the fisherman, "now we can enjoy ourselves."

"Yes," said the wife, "we're going to enjoy it."

Everything went well for about a week or two, and then the wife said, "Listen, husband, the hut is much too cramped, and the yard and garden are too little. I want a large stone castle. Go back to the flounder and tell him to give us a castle."

"Ah, wife," said the husband. "The flounder has just given us a hut, and I don't want to go back again so soon. The flounder might be unwilling to do anything."

*"What do you mean?" said the wife. "He can easily do it, and he'll be glad to do it. Just go back to him!" So the fisherman left, and his heart grew heavy. When he got to the sea, the water was purple, dark blue,
gray, and dense but still calm. Then he stood there and said:*

"Flounder, flounder, in the sea,
if you're a man, then speak to me.
Though I don't agree with my wife's request,
I've come to ask it nonetheless."

"What now! What does she want?" the flounder asked.

"Oh," said the fisherman, somewhat distressed. "My wife wants to live in a large stone castle."

"Go home. She's standing in front of the door," the flounder said. The fisherman went home, and his wife was standing in front of a large palace

"So, husband," she said, "isn't this beautiful?"

He went inside with her, and there were many servants, and the walls were all bright. The chairs and tables were made of gold. Behind the palace was a huge yard and a park half a mile long with deer and does and rabbits. There was also a stable for cows and horses.

"Oh," said the husband, "now let's live in the beautiful castle and be content."

"We'll have to think about that," said the wife, "and sleep on it." Then they went to bed. The next morning the wife woke up. It was just daybreak, and he poked her husband in his side with her elbow and said, "Husband, get up. We must be king and rule this entire country."

"Ah, wife!" said the husband. "Why should we be king? I don't want to be king."

"Well," said the wife, "then I'll be king."

"Oh, wife," said the husband, "where can you be king? The flounder won't want to make you king."

"Husband," said the wife, "go straight to him and tell him I must be king!"

The fisherman went but was very distressed that his wife wanted to be king.

When he got to the sea, it was completely gray and black, and the water was fermenting from below. The fisherman stood there and said:

"Flounder, flounder, in the sea,
if you're a man, then speak to me.
Though I don't agree with my wife's request,
I've come to ask it nonetheless."

"Well, what does she want?" asked the flounder.

"Oh," said the man, "she wants to be king."

"Go back home," said the flounder. "She's already king."

Then the man went home, and as he approached the palace, he saw that there were many soldiers, drums, and trumpets. His wife was sitting on a high throne of gold and diamonds, and she wore a large golden crown. Two rows of ladies-in-waiting were standing on either side of her, each lady a head shorter than the next.

"Oh," said the fisherman, "now you're king, aren't you?"

"Yes," said his wife, "I am king." After he gazed at her for some time, he said, "Oh, wife, it's wonderful that you're king! Now let's not wish for anything more."

"No, husband," the wife said as she became very restless. "I have too much time on my hands, and I can't stand it anymore. I'm king, but now I also want to be emperor."

"Oh, wife," said the fisherman, "why do you want to be emperor?"

"Husband," she said, "go to the flounder. I want to be emperor!'

"Oh, wife," the husband said. "He can't make you emperor. I don't want to tell that to the flounder."

"I'm king," she said, "and you're just my husband. Go there at once!"

The fisherman went away, but as he was walking, he thought, "This won't turn out well at all. It's outrageous for her to be emperor. The flounder's going to become sick and tired of this in the end." When he got to the sea, it was all black and dense, and a strong wind whipped across the surface and made the water curdle. Then the fisherman stepped forward and said:

"Flounder, flounder, in the sea,
if you're a man, then speak to me.
Though I don't agree with my wife's request,
I've come to ask it nonetheless."

"Well, what does she want?" asked the flounder.

"Oh, flounder," he said. "My wife wants to be emperor."

"Go back home," said the flounder. "She's already emperor."

Then the man went home, and when he arrived, he saw his wife sitting on a very high throne made from a single piece of gold. She was wearing a large crown three yards tall and covered with diamonds and garnets. She was flanked on either side by two rows of bodyguards, each man shorter than the next, beginning with a tremendous giant two miles tall and ending with the tiniest dwarf, who was no bigger than my pinky. There were also many princes and dukes standing before her, and her husband stepped up and said, "Wife, now you're emperor, aren't you?"

"Yes," she said, "I'm emperor."

"Oh," said the fisherman, and he gazed at her for some time, "it's wonderful that you're emperor."

"Husband," she replied. "why are you standing there like that? I'm emperor, but now I also want to be pope."

"Oh, wife," said the husband. "Why do you want to be pope?"

"Husband," she said. "I want to be pope!"

"No, wife," said the fisherman. "The flounder can't make you pope. It won't turn out well."

"Stop talking nonsense, husband!" said the wife. "If he can make me emperor, he can also make me pope. Go there at once!"

So the fisherman went off, but he felt rather queasy. He was trembling, and his knees began to wobble. A strong wind swept across the land. The water rose up in waves, and the waves splashed against the shore. Ships were in distress as they were tossed up and down by the waves. Though there was still a little blue in the middle of the sky, the horizon was completely red, as if a heavy thunderstorm were coming. Then he stepped forward and said:

"Flounder, flounder, in the sea
if you're a man, then speak to me.
Though I don't agree with my wife's request,
I've come to ask it nonetheless."

"Well, what does she want?" asked the flounder.

"Oh," the man said, "she wants to be pope."

"Go back home," said the flounder. "She's already pope."

Then the man went home, and when he arrived, his wife was sitting on a throne two miles high and was wearing three large golden crowns on her head. Numerous bishops and priests were standing around her, and there were two rows of candles on either side of her. The biggest candle was as thick and as large as the highest tower, and the tiniest was a church candle.

"Wife," the man said as he took a good look at her, "are you the pope?"

"Yes," she said, "I'm pope."

"Oh, wife," he said, "Isn't it wonderful that you're pope. You must be satisfied. Now that you're pope, you can't become anything greater."

"I'll think about it," said the wife.

Then they both went to bed, but she wasn't satisfied, and her ambition prevented her from sleeping. She kept thinking of ways she might become greater than she was. When the sun began to rise, she sat at the window and thought, "Aha, I could also make the sun rise!" Then she became quite grim and poked her husband and said, "Husband, go to the flounder. I want to be like God."

The husband was still half asleep, but he was so shocked by what she had said that he fell out of the bed.

"Ah, wife," he said. "Be content and remain pope."

"No," his wife said. "I won't have any peace of mind and won't be able bear it until I can make the sun and moon rise. I want to be like God!"

"Ahh, wife!" the husband said. "The flounder can't do that. He can make you emperor and pope, but he can't make you God."

"Husband," she said and looked ghastly, "I want to be like God. I want you to go to the flounder at once!"

Now his limbs began to tremble, and he was filled with fear. Outside a great storm was raging so much that all the trees and mountains were shaking. The sky was pitch black, and there was thunder and lightning. Black waves rose up in the sea as high as mountains, and they all had crests of white foam on top. Then the fisherman said:

"Flounder, flounder, in the sea,
if you're a man, then speak to me.
Though I don't agree with my wife's request,
I've come to ask it nonetheless."

"Well, what does she want?" the flounder asked.
"Oh," he said, "she wants to be like God."
"Go back home. She's sitting in your piss pot again.
And that's where they are still sitting this very day.

***

What I refer to as the domination knot is the intertwining of different threads that support and sustain each other, several of which are invisible but whose interconnectedness keeps capitalist society running. Intertwined in this knot are: the profit-driven actions of capital that incorporate living labour in the form of wage labour, thereby always further developing the productive forces, thereby depleting and cutting back on labour, which is its source—this is already a complex dialectical connection. Then there are the invisible, unspoken, and historyless deeds that are all necessary to restore the lives of people and the nature surrounding them. These form a strand, have a different temporal logic, are difficult to rationalize—that is, make more efficient and faster—in order to be profitable: the loving mother, the heroic nurse, the charity volunteer worker, and the environmentalist are in this context just as well-known as the catastrophes that attack people from behind, from the brutalization and degeneration of entire generations and sections of the population to the uninhabitability of the earth. Many of these activities remain invisible—*Readers Digest* used to have a column, "People Never Forgotten," dedicated to such acts of humanity that were undertaken voluntarily and without self-serving benefit—and many have been transformed into wage labour in developed capitalist countries, where they have a tolerated, poor, and poorly paid reputation.

Within this interlocking, the neglect of people themselves as human beings goes almost unmentioned—development is elitist, something that only the rich can afford, while the urge to develop what is humanly possible is stifled in the consumer frenzy, which is also a basis for growth, consumption, etc., and has taken advantage of the desire of the fisherman's wife in a different way, both tamed and significantly more transient. And it also goes unnoticed that people are kept subaltern in immaturity regarding the shaping of society—what we call politics. These four threads are intricately interwoven, secured, and developed and can be found in our habits, actions, morals, hopes, desires, and common sense (to merge = four-in-one perspective).[3]

Brecht sums it up:

> Some people have got the wrong end of the stick about rules, and what ruling is. Most people live their whole lives without realizing they're being ruled, and that's a fact. They think they're doing whatever they'd be doing if there were no authorities or any other kind of ruler.[4]

Brecht's character, Kalle, in *Refugee Conversations*, is succinctly saying that rule needs the ruled, who practically confirm their rule day and night.[5]

One can imagine the interaction of these diverse forces, as well as how enormous the field of research and practice is that must be explored to liberate oneself from domination, and how many must change themselves and their conditions.

Gramsci speaks of the task:

> it is necessary to elaborate a doctrine in which these relations are seen as active and in movement, establishing quite clearly that the source of this activity is the consciousness of the individual man who knows, wishes, admires, creates (in so far as he does know, wish, admire, create, etc) and conceives of himself not as isolated but rich in the possibilities offered him by other men and by the society of things of which he cannot help having a certain knowledge.[6]

However, what is the point of speaking of a domination knot in this context rather than simply of interaction?

I turn to the metaphor of shoelaces. Everyone knows that two threads are tied together so that they cannot easily unravel on their own. To guarantee this, you tie a double knot. If you have four or more threads, it becomes almost impossible—like the Gordian knot—and the solution remains the task. But, and this is the important point here, there is always the possibility of pulling on the wrong end, thereby tightening the knot and making the solution impossible.

In the project of the Four-In-One Perspective (which is certainly well known here and is seeking, and has even occasionally found, acceptance in some quarters of the left), the idea of the knot and its insidious way of tightening as it is being untied is fundamental. This is easy to understand and explain when considering the pressures during the "Great Crisis" if one looks at labour trapped in the wage form and its reduction as an exclusive policy. The neglect of all other labour in society is just as evident as the fact that the target group becomes smaller and smaller as the productive forces develop. On the other hand, many other jobs are gradually disappearing from view, while their wage-based components are falling victim to the austerity measures of the crisis—as is happening in the healthcare system, school system, and social and youth work. Conversely, many care and reproductive forms of labour are generally in great need, as there is not enough time for them. Therefore, the struggles for them must be conducted differently than only through a reduction in working hours. However, if one starts to pull on this thread and, for example, demands childcare allowance, parental allowance, maternity allowance, and thus wholly converts this area into the wage form, one quickly learns that reactionary images of motherhood are almost inevitably pursued, which, as Bloch puts it, nail the female sex "to the cross of history" forever.[7] This—pulled alone—is the wrong end. The knot must be untied differently. Leaving the tangle of knots as they are and carefully pulling at the thread of all-round development consolidates the boundaries that have been drawn around the training of elites, because the connection with economic growth leads to support for those who are economically useful, which neither benefits the all-round development of the personality, nor the development of all senses, but, as is evident, leads to a concentration on the inventiveness of what is feasible, as far as the domination and use of nature is concerned. The prolongation of life for the rich, replacement of their organs with stolen ones from elsewhere, flawless children for some…etc. One must, as Donna Haraway demands, compile a list of inventions and developments that promote the exclusion of many from general humanity, thus supporting domination.[8] Finally, politics. All improvements in political representation, which are certainly necessary, push into the background the need for grassroots politics—socialist democracy, in which everyone is empowered to take the shaping of society into their own hands.

Although this sounds unbearably rhetorical, because we no longer believe that it could succeed, it remains a long-term goal; our policy remains the deepening of democracy as an action taken by everyone. Not a reduction in working hours for full employment and growth, but its reduction so that I have more time for fairytales, for other people, for politics, which I consider essential. Sometimes I bring everything together.

The question remains why people are not fighting back in the current major crisis, but are instead mostly electing those who caused this crisis as their representatives. Posing the question in more general terms reveals the answer. The glue that belongs to the tightening threads of the domination knot is that the reinforcements also contain rewards. A laced shoe makes walking easier. Every form of domination involves not only habit but, with it, also the agency of the subjected. This makes it even more challenging to encourage individuals to change their living conditions. There is no holding on without support. The solution to the domination knot is, therefore, not only incredibly long-term and complicated work—but also it is one that must be tackled in all areas simultaneously and requires everyone's energy and time.

Everyone is pulling on the individual strands. They are loosening their grip on full-time employment and want to spend less time there in order to devote the freed-up time to caring work and kindness in the world. They recalibrate; some no longer consider wage labour the exclusive center of their lives, others do not want to devote all their time to domestic matters, but both recognize that in greater leisure, human senses accomplish more, are more enjoyable, even if still strenuous, than mere toil in one form or another. With a sigh of relief, they look around, see that there is little that is right, and also realize that they must work together to shape society, that is, take politics into their own hands. In these four simultaneous movements, the knots loosen, and domination becomes unstable. This loosening is anti-capitalist and radically democratic, thus systematic resistance is to be expected.

Finally, Brecht, who provides intellectual gymnastics for the mind and is an excellent political teacher, even if we can no longer fully share his comprehensive hope:

> When the ruling class loses its grip, the ruled usually collapse at first. The institutions are already faltering and crumbling, and the oppressed are far from showing any signs of taking over. Against them stands their religion, their art of living, which they have learned with difficulty, much of it from the enemy, some of it in battle with the enemy, a complex set of habits and maxims. Therefore, the revolution must have something business-like, an organised enterprise in which they can recognise features of their everyday life, in short, sensible, to involve the masses.[9]

Addendum: Let us return to the fisherman's wife, who sat idle in a hovel at the story's beginning while harboring higher wishes. The one-sided image, forgetting her actions, is necessary to downplay wishes in general, especially female ones. She should stay in the hovel and do what is necessary without any further complaint. So, it can be assumed that humanity will survive for the time being and that progress lies in the hands of the fisherman. However, he will not come up with better, more profitable use of his labour-power on his own—so the wish must be placed in the right hands, which can then, in turn, make use of the fisherman as available labour power in an increasingly social, that is, cooperative, form based in the division of labour. The control over women's bodies and labour remains unmentioned—a force that falls prey to knots. It is, therefore, also important and part of the domination knot that a large part of society's labour is unrecognized, unconscious, and hidden. The knot thus takes a form that is harder to decipher. Untying it requires insight and, with it, a perception that juxtaposes the forms of labour so that they are simultaneously visible, and only from there can a narrative for the future be written, and its step-by-step realization begun.

Notes

1 Editors' Note: This lecture was delivered at a symposium hosted by the *Rosa Luxemburg Foundation* in honour of Frigga Haug's 75th birthday.

2 Editors' Note: We have included the full text of "The Fisherman and his Wife" fairytale by the Grimm Brothers, to provide readers with context for Haug's essay, which reference the tale. Brothers Grimm, "The Fisherman and his Wife," *The Original Folk & Fairy Tales of the Brothers Grimm*, trans. Jack Zipes (Princeton University Press, 2014) 56–62.

3 This perspective is outlined in more detail in Frigga Haug's essay "Four-in-One," included in this volume.

4 Bertolt Brecht, "Flüchtlingsgespräche," *Prosa 4*, *Gesammelte Werke 14* (Suhrkamp, 1967), 1437; Bertolt Brecht, *Refugee Conversations*, trans. Romy Fursland and ed. Tom Kuhn (Methuen Drama, 2019), 46.

5 Translator's Note: In Brecht's incomplete comic satire, *Refugee Conversations,* two characters, the intellectual Ziffel and worker Kalle discuss the experiences of refugees from Nazi Germany, highlighting the absurdity of bureaucracy and the failings of host societies. The play was written in the early 1940s, during the Second World War, and explores the lives of those expelled from Germany.

6 Antonio Gramsci, "Philosophie der Praxis," *Gefängnishefte*, *Band 6*, Heft 10, § 54, ed. Klaus Bochmann and Wolfgang Fritz Haug (Argument, 1994), 1349; Antonio Gramsci, *Selections from the Prison Notebooks* (International Publishers 1971), 353–4.

7 Ernst Bloch, *Tendenz – Latenz – Utopie*, Ergänzungsband zur Gesamtausgabe (Suhrkamp, 1978).

8 Donna Haraway, "Lieber Cyborg als Göttin," *Monströse Versprechen. Die Gender- und Technologie-Essays* (Argument Verlag, 1995), 165–184; Donna Haraway, "A Manifesto for Cyborgs: Science, Technology, and Socialist-Feminism in the 1980s," *Socialist Review*, no. 80 (1985): 65–108.

9 Bertolt Brecht, "Marxistische Studien," *Schriften zur Politik und Gesellschaft*, *Gesammelte Werke 20* (Suhrkamp, 1967), 120.

References

Brecht, Bertolt. "Flüchtlingsgespräche." In *Prosa 4, Gesammelte Werke 14*. Suhrkamp, 1967a.

Brecht, Bertolt. "Marxistische Studien." In *Schriften zur Politik und Gesellschaft, Gesammelte Werke 20*. Suhrkamp, 1967b.

Brecht, Bertolt. *Refugee Conversations*. Translated by Romy Fursland and edited by Tom Kuhn. Methuen Drama, 2019.

Brothers Grimm. "The Fisherman and his Wife." In *The Original Folk & Fairy Tales of the Brothers Grimm*. Translated by Jack Zipes. Princeton University Press, 2014.

Bloch, Ernst. *Tendenz – Latenz – Utopie.* Ergänzungsband zur Gesamtausgabe. Suhrkamp, 1978.

Gramsci, Antonio. *Selections from the Prison Notebooks*. International Publishers, 1971.
Gramsci, Antonio. "Philosophie der Praxis." In *Gefängnishefte, Band 6*. Edited by Klaus Bochmann and Wolfgang Fritz Haug. Argument, 1994.
Haraway, Donna. "Lieber Cyborg als Göttin." In *Monströse Versprechen. Die Gender-und Technologie-Essays,* 165–184. Argument Verlag, 1995.
Haraway, Donna. "A Manifesto for Cyborgs: Science, Technology, and Socialist-Feminism in the 1980s." *Socialist Review* 80 (1985): 65–108.

Chapter 13

The Four-in-One-Perspective

A Utopia by Women, A Utopia for All[1]

Frigga Haug

The following considerations concern justice in the distribution of wage labour, housework, community work, and development opportunities. For a long time, political projects in these four areas have been pursued separately. The purpose of this text is to provide a compass that orients these various projects toward a common framework, which, by linking them, becomes truly critical, even revolutionary, whereas each taken individually tends to fizzle out sooner or later.

Among the fairy tales by the Brothers Grimm, one tells the story of a pretty but lazy girl who refuses to work at the spinning wheel. Her mother finally loses her temper. She gives the girl a good beating. The Queen, who happens to be passing by, hears her screaming. She stops and asks the mother why she is beating her daughter. The mother is not ashamed of beating her but instead of having to reveal her daughter's laziness. So, she cunningly lies, immediately spotlighting her poverty, "I cannot stop her from spinning; she wants to spin forever and ever, and I am poor and cannot provide the flax." This awakens the Queen's desire for such an industrious worker, and she takes the girl to the castle. There, she leads the girl to three chambers full of flax to be spun and even promises her eldest son as a husband, since now it is not her poverty that counts but "unflagging diligence is dowry enough." The Queen's son spends his time dancing and singing, playing music and writing poetry, painting, acting, riding, travelling, fencing, and hunting, as befits a King's son. The girl, however, is not only lazy, but she cannot spin at all. When the Queen returns three days later to inspect the results of the work, she finds that the girl has accomplished nothing. The girl apologizes, claiming she is too sad to work because of the distance from her mother's house. The Queen is touched but urges her to begin at last. Left alone again with the flax, the girl gazes helplessly out the window. Three ugly women are walking down on the street. The first has a clubfoot, the second has a drooping lower lip, and the third has a thumb three fingers wide. They promise to spin the flax if she will invite them to the wedding, exhibit no shame in knowing them, but instead call them her aunts and allow them to sit beside her and share in the wedding feast. The girl agrees, and the three women immediately set to work, and before long, they have beautifully spun all the flax, leaving the chambers empty.

DOI: 10.4324/9781003480143-13

The Queen is as pleased as the eldest son, who is to marry such a hardworking and skilled wife, and the wedding is arranged. The girl asks that her three aunts be invited. As the three overworked women step through the door, the groom cries out in alarm: "How do you come by such nasty friends?" He then asks the first one, "How did you get such a broad foot?" "From pedaling the spinning wheel," she replies, "from pedaling." The groom then asks the second: "How did you get that dropping lip?" "From licking the thread," she answers, "from licking." He then asks the third: "How did you get that broad thumb?" "From spinning the thread," she replies, "from spinning the thread." The prince becomes frightened and declares: "Now never again shall my beautiful bride touch a spinning wheel." And so, the girl is freed from the harmful task of spinning flax. The pact has paid off twice for her: she gets the prince and is spared the work of spinning. Now she, too, can devote herself to luxury, beauty, the leisurely activities, and arts that, after all, are more befitting of a Queen.

There is more to the story than meets the eye. It tells of female cunning, of hard labour and poverty, of strange shame, of a life of wealth attained by birth or, in the case of women, through marriage. It initially draws us into agreeing to ally ourselves with the mother, outraged by the daughter's laziness. Yet soon we, too, find that resistance to work is justified. Since we at least have an inkling that one-sided and possibly lifelong wear and tear from work can lead to disfigurement and premature exhaustion, we now spontaneously, albeit somewhat hesitantly, ally ourselves against work, because we cannot afford a life of luxury without work for ourselves or our children. And yet, we are tempted by the prospect of not only being allowed to be lazy but also of having every opportunity to develop our cultural abilities and enjoy something like leisurely learning. In short, we become, for the time being, imaginary members of that part of the ruling class that is itself exempt even from the labour of domination, in which individuals develop at the expense of the majority of the population, who, as a result, lead a stunted life with regard to human potential. We suddenly realize that, out of sheer habit, we have come to accept that there are hardly any opportunities for development for most people.

For all the cruelty it proclaims, the fairytale world is full of dreams of a desirable life. For our purposes, we do not turn to dreams such as those of the land of plenty, where milk and honey flow endlessly, and roasted pigs with knives and forks in their backs lie ready to be eaten. In such visions, the connection to our active lives is completely severed. Instead, we turn to considerations that, although utopian, are potentially still operating in our world, and upon which they urge change.

From Ernst Bloch, we learned to draw strength for change from utopias. If actual history is a history of the oppression of the many, the power for change retreats into dream images of a society without alienation. If we are stuck in the present in such a way that change is difficult to imagine, and yet we still dream of it, we should bring the dream back to the ground of reality. Bloch calls such longing "the only honest quality of human beings," and a "hidden homesickness" that feeds on the "preconscious" and the not-yet.[2] It is about crossing boundaries, about planning better conditions that would be possible, in other words, about making utopia more concrete.[3] And finally, it is about taking seriously what was already conscious in the French Revolution: freedom, equality, fraternity—which we as women translate as solidarity and supplement with justice.

That one harbors curiosity about the future, regains concrete possibilities, and recognizes what is to come as an explosive force in the present—this is the sense in which we use utopian thinking.

In the fairytale we playfully saw dimensions of life between which one could choose: labour and, in contrast to it, even if rarely practised, luxury, not as laziness but also as an activity, as the development of creative possibilities. However, one does not disappear from the sphere of human necessity if, like the daughter, one can simply choose the other. It is accomplished through the division of labour, or rather, the division of labour also appears as some enjoying what others produce, developing at the expense of others. To divide labour as in the aforementioned fairytale, the division of labour must be linked to domination. The division of labour and the control of some over others also applies to the relationship between men and women—as the first class relation, as Marx and Engels put it—and then to that between head and hand, between city and country. The history of the division of labour, its blessings and curses, must be studied separately—here we consider only the result: the control of men over the labour of women, of owners of capital over those who work for wages, of rulers over the ruled subalterns, who do not create their own society, the development of some at the expense of many.

The protest movements, born of such inequalities, from which we wish to learn, entered history at different times and protested, in part, against the various forms of oppression that most afflicted the oppressed. Here, we focus on four such impulses for change: those arising from wage labour as labour commanded by others; those that stem from men's control over women; those arising from the separation of politics from the disenfranchised subalterns; and finally, those that protest against the fact that most people are denied the concrete possibility of developing their potential. The various impulses interact, determine, and shape one another; they must therefore always be studied in relation to one another.

The labour movement arose from the form of wage labour with the aim of liberating all people from bondage, because there could be no other class below those who own only their labour power. The aim of liberation was directed at all people since, by and large, everyone was considered a wage labourer, at least as a possibility. The labour movement had the most important theorists, who could leave behind a manifesto outlining what should be done. This gave rise to a profound willingness on the part of the representatives of this movement to consider themselves the sole center. Women's liberation was accordingly considered in this context. Engels writes:

> The emancipation of women becomes possible only when women are enabled to take part in production on a large, social scale, and when domestic duties require their attention only to a minor degree…which not only permits of the

> participation of women in production in large numbers, but actually calls for it and, moreover, strives more and more to reduce private domestic duties to a public industry.[4]

And Rosa Luxemburg:

> As a bourgeois woman, the female is a parasite on society; her function consists in sharing in the consumption of the fruits of exploitation. As a petty-bourgeois woman, she is a workhorse for the family. As a modern female proletarian, the woman becomes a human being for the first time, *since the [proletarian] struggle is the first to prepare human beings to make a contribution to culture, to the history of humanity.*[5]

Even more radically, Lenin writes with regard to peasant women and proletarian women:

> Notwithstanding all the laws emancipating woman, she continues to be a domestic slave, because petty housework crushes, strangles, stultifies and degrades her, chains her to the kitchen and the nursery, and she wastes her labour on barbarously unproductive, petty, nerve-racking, stultifying and crushing drudgery.[6]

The women's movements, especially those of the 1970s, revealed that this view, not only regarded housework and care work negatively, as something that should be abolished rather than also as a place where local knowledge and corresponding attitudes that are indispensable to humanity (situated knowledge) can be gained, but also that a critique of wage labour is not enough to solve everything, that further domination must be dismantled: that of male control over female labour through confinement in the home, sexual control even to the point of violence, exclusion from all decision-making positions, lower pay once the usually necessary additional wage labour has been taken on—most of which persists to this day and is ideologically secured, for example, by the claim that happiness essentially lies in the family, that the development of children lies with the mother, and so on.

The protest from women's groups was both more one-sided and more comprehensive than that of the labour movement. Mariarosa Dalla Costa linked women's oppression to the function of unpaid housework in the reproduction of capitalist social relations.[7] She called on women to "defend themselves against the unpaid housework, and suppression of their sexuality, and the separation of the family from the outside world."[8] She called for a housewives' strike; women had worked enough and should "reject the myth of liberation through work."[9]

And Anke Wolf-Graaf comprehensively states that,

> Reproductive labour is the invisible basis...upon which the entire pyramid of capitalist accumulation rests.[10]

Precisely because a standpoint was adopted that did not identify class domination as the sole source of oppression and exploitation, and therefore also of liberation, other dimensions of daily life came to light. Women insisted that unwaged labour should not only be recognized and made socially visible—they also demonstrated that it was precisely in this area of reproductive labour that qualities and forms indispensable to a humane society were being developed. They scandalized the fact that there is a massive amount of work other than wage labour in society that is done by women; that there is another form of control besides that over labour power in the public sphere, namely that which exists in the private sphere, which is exerted through bodies, both sexually and through violence; that privacy is not merely confinement but also exclusion from social spheres—in this way, aiming for liberation became more comprehensive, more radical. And it was precisely this widespread exclusion from socially relevant spheres that unleashed a desire to participate in shaping society, to no longer see politics as a matter for those above, for others, to reject representation, to develop the aim of taking one's own destiny and thus that of all people into one's own hands. "Liberation cannot be handed to us, we have to conquer it ourselves. If we fail to conquer it ourselves, then it will have no consequences for us," writes Peter Weiß in *The Aesthetics of Resistance*.[11] This also applies to women.

Although the denial of opportunities for development affects most members of society, it was the women's perspective that truly radically and publicly scandalized it. Precisely because education and the arts were accessible to children of the bourgeoisie, provided they were male, the daughters of bourgeoisie were the first to see what had been denied them. Virginia Woolf sharply describes the situation of bourgeois women in the first women's movement (in *The Three Guineas*), showing how the struggle for equality cannot aim at equality but is, from the very beginning, even in the bourgeois women's movement, a transgression toward a utopia that does not yet know itself.

A progressive, educated man asks a woman with a feminine education (in literature, some piano playing, etc.) to help him prevent the impending war. In examining the question, she explores all relevant areas—the non-participation of everyone in politics, including in preventing wars; the ideological alignment with war through patriotism, which she does not see in her daughters; the impossibility of making a significant impact on society due to a lack of education and a profession; and, at the same time, the criticism of the traditional educational content and forms for men, as well as of wage labour and corresponding training. Virginia Woolf, based on the situation of women, designs a utopian model for a different kind of education: the college for women teachers

> must teach only the arts that can be taught cheaply and practices by poor people; such as, medicine, mathematics, music, painting, and literature. It should teach the arts of human intercourse; the art of understanding other people's lives and

> minds, and the little arts of talk, of dress, of cookery that are allied with them. The aim of the new college, the cheap college, should not be to segregate and specialize, but to combine. It should explore the ways in which mind and body can be made to co-operate; discover what new combinations make good wholes in human life.[12]

The solution necessarily aims at a different society in which women can also be human, which presupposes the humanity of men.

Since Virginia Woolf, that is, since the 1930s, the situation of women has improved in many ways. Education and access to professions are also available to women; even within the government, there is debate about how to reconcile work and family life, albeit almost exclusively for women rather than for men; above all, the productive forces of labour—the transferring of work to machines, the development of computer technology—have advanced so far that the necessary labour time people need to devote to earning the necessities of life has shrunk to a fraction of what it used to be.

It is high time to formulate our utopia more precisely as an orienting yearning and a political compass.

In the fairy tale I spoke of at the beginning, no one would have advocated expanding and generalizing spinning labour that disfigures bodies as much as possible—on the contrary, it was utopian, in the good sense, to abolish the lifelong fixation on a partial function because:

> It converts the labourer into a crippled monstrosity, by forcing his detail dexterity at the expense of a world of productive capabilities and instincts.[13]

Thus, the possible progress was also to be seen as in such a development of the productive forces that would allow working hours to be shortened and the "realm of necessity" to be pushed back in order to develop human essential powers in the "realm of freedom"—as Marx again puts it.[14] In the meantime, the amount of work necessary for mere survival has indeed decreased dramatically; yet, the freed-up time is not used for development, but turns against workers in the form of unemployment. This leads to the call to "create work," which, taken literally, is absurd; rewarding those who promise to "create jobs." This promise is silent about its prerequisites. It sounds as if income is being created where none exists, or as if the affected people are languishing in the jungles of Hartz IV.[15] From one of the perspectives of women, such promises as "creating additional jobs" must sound perverse from the outset. One can hardly finish all the overwork that results from organizing what we call reproductive labour (on oneself, on children, on men who work full-time, on the elderly, the sick, friends, neighbors, etc.) while simultaneously working part-time—where calls for personal development, learning, theatre, culture, enjoyment, and a good life sound quite cynical and political participation that influences the whole is unthinkable.

We conclude that in all this, in over-burdening and under-challenging, in overwork and unemployment, in restlessness and waiting, a profound, general injustice prevails. It affects the division of labour in society and, within it, the space and time for the development of that very society and the people within it.

Therefore, as a prospective guideline for future politics, we propose a fundamental change in the division of labour. What we are aiming for is to connect these four areas of human activity:

1 Work for the necessary means of subsistence in the form of wage labour.
2 Work on oneself and other people, what we are accustomed to calling "humanity"—for as Marx recognized, with Charles Fourier, the "degree of emancipation of woman is the natural measure of general emancipation"[16] because "in the relation of woman to man, of the weak to the strong, the victory of human nature over brutality is most evident,"[17] because even if the weaker can grow to the same extent, the truly human reveals itself, which also includes love; or, once again in Marx's words,

> [t]he direct, natural, and necessary relation of person to person is the relation of man to woman. In this relationship, therefore, is sensuously manifested, reduced to an observable fact, the extent to which the human essence has become nature to man, or to which nature to him has become the human essence of man.[18]

3 Third, it is about developing dormant potential, developing through lifelong learning, enjoying life not merely as a consumer but as an active participant, and thus being able to develop a different idea of the good life.
4 And finally, it is about the overarching need for us to take the time to intervene in shaping society, that is, to become politically active.

First, the politics of labour, its quality, duration, time, and remuneration can build on the experience in the movements associated with labour.

Second, the question of working on the next generation, on all others, and on oneself, commonly referred to as reproductive labour, brings together a critique of patriarchy by fighting for this space of human development for all genders.

Third, the time needed for personal development, clashes with the politics of the time regime in our way of life, in which we must, therefore, as fourth, intervene and put the representative model of politics in its place.

This is the outline of a more comprehensive concept of justice that women can formulate, one that begins with the division of labour and the associated expenditure of time. If we assume that each person can contribute approximately 16 hours a day to the total social labour, it immediately becomes clear that talk of crisis because we are running out of labour is based on an extremely restrictive concept of labour and wants to cling to it whatever the cost. The situation looks radically different from the perspective of life as a whole and its human administration.

In labour politics, the guiding principle is the necessary reduction of working hours for everyone to a quarter of the time actively used, that is, to four hours—in the long term, this will solve the problems of unemployment (we will then have fewer people than jobs), along with precarious employment and temporary work. In other words, everyone will work part-time, or rather, the term itself will no longer have any meaningful significance, and we will be able to focus on the quality of work, demanding that it corresponds to human abilities and potentials.

The politics surrounding basic income are also becoming more life-affirming. Since everyone has the right to four hours of waged labour, and this is then also available, the question of whether basic income is unconditional can no longer be raised. Instead, it goes without saying that all individuals have sufficient income to live on and are equally active in each of the four areas: in wage labour, in caring for themselves and others, in developing their dormant potential, and, finally, in political and social engagement. This can also be expressed by saying that every person is enabled to organize their life so that they spend four hours a day in each of these areas. This is not to be understood dogmatically, as if one had to go from one area to another with a punch clock in hand, no longer feeling sufficiently at home in any of them. Rather, as soon as one begins to grasp one's lifestyle in these dimensions, one will quickly notice that the boundaries are not fixed, that the areas permeate one another and are intrinsically connected. The division of four four-hour periods is a model that, like a compass, can decisively orient strategies for change. Incidentally, the shame repeatedly invoked at the beginning of the fairy tale is dispelled by the obligation to oneself and others to actually engage in such diverse human activities.

For reproductive family labour, this means, first and foremost, a generalization. Just as no one can be excluded from wage labour, neither can they be excluded from reproductive labour—all people, men and women alike, can and should develop their social human skills in this area. This settles the dispute over childcare benefits without devaluing the quality of labour done here; indeed, on the contrary, only now, through generalization rather than assignment solely to women and mothers, can the general claim be realized that this labour is skilled and must, therefore be learned like any other work. The many reports of abused and neglected children bear eloquent witness to this.

In a conversation with fathers who shared general concerns about their sons' development, caught between refusal, drugs, violence, and despair, I listened with interest as they told me that civil services in a hospital intensive care unit and in geriatric care had brought about a boost of humanization: instead of cynicism, a sense of purpose in life had emerged. Why not include civil service for all in the social education program?

The question of individual development is about the possibility of seizing diverse possibilities inherent in human beings from the very beginning, regardless of gender, class, or skin color—processes that continue through life. Or, to put it another way: it should no longer be acceptable for some to speak multiple languages, compose music, write poetry, paint, and travel, like Goethe, continuing to perfect themselves, while others have to be content if they can read and write at all.

Our political aspiration boils down to the fact that shaping society should not be a specialized task divided between groups, with some engaging in politics while others, the vast majority, suffer the consequences. The Zapatista women can serve as a model for us here. As the poorest of the poor, they insisted, as a matter of course, that the unconditional protection of indigenous culture cannot be a demand made by women, as liberal U.N. policies proposed, because violence against women is inscribed within it. Instead, women need the right to practical participation in all political decisions and to reject any customs that violate their physical or mental dignity. In return, they demand half the votes in all political decision-making bodies. This also applies to healthcare, medical competence for all, co-decision making in schools, the selection of teachers, the quality of production facilities, the development of infrastructure, knowledge about contraception, and universal access to information and learning. Their goal is to banish violence from everyday life.[19]

Prospectively, it is about creating society from the bottom up: as Rosa Luxemburg said of democracy, it must

> proceed step by step out of the active participation of the masses; it must be under their direct influence, subjected to the control of complete public activity; it must arise out of the growing political training of the mass of people.[20]

One could now set about pursuing the four areas of wage labour, reproductive work, political work, and individual development separately, and in turn treat this as a division of labour in which individual groups, parties, or even currents within parties each occupy an isolated area as their trademark. Class-conscious, some pursue labour politics that that can benefit workers; others seek a perspective from the past, a backward-looking utopia for mothers that nails us women alive to the cross of history, as Bloch puts it[21]; the third group focuses on developing an elite, an elite that demonstrates human capabilities in an Olympic-worthy manner; the fourth group pursues participatory political models in non-essential areas, such as turning television into a model institution for viewers' wishes, involving the workforce in organizing Christmas celebrations, encouraging the population to recycle, etc. In all cases, one will experience that each area, when made the focus of politics, can become downright reactionary.

The art of politics lies in the interconnection of the four areas. None should be pursued without the others, aiming for a politics and at the same time a way of life that would be comprehensive, vibrant, meaningful, impactful, and enjoyable. This is not a short-term goal, nor is it achievable here and now; however, it can serve as a compass for setting short-term goals in politics, as a benchmark for our demands, as the basis for our critique, as hope, as a concrete utopia that includes all people and in which the development of each individual can finally become a prerequisite for the development of all.

Notes

1 Editors' Note: This text is an excerpt from a more extensive work by Frigga Haug. See Frigga Haug, *Die Vier-in-einem-Perspektive: Politik von Frauen für eine neue Linke* (Argument Verlag, 2008), particularly 13–23.
2 Ernst Bloch, *Tendenz – Latenz – Utopie*, Ergänzungsband zur Gesamtausgabe (Suhrkamp, 1978), 55, 288.
3 Bloch, *Tendenz – Latenz – Utopie*, 290.
4 Friedrich Engels, "Der Ursprung der Familie, des Privateigentums und des Staats," *Marx Engels Werke Band 21* (Dietz, 1962), 25–173, 158; Frederick Engels, "The Origin of the Family, Private Property and the State," *Marx and Engels Collected Works, Volume 26: Engels 1882–89* (International Publishers, 1976), 126–276, 262.
5 Rosa Luxemburg, "Die Proletarierin," *Gesammelte Werke Band 3: 3. Juli 1911 bis Juli 1914* (Dietz, 2002), 410; Rosa Luxemburg, "The Proletarian Woman," *The Rosa Luxemburg Reader*, ed. Peter Hudis and Kevin B. Anderson (Monthly Review Press, 2004), 243.
6 Vladimir Iljitsch Lenin, *Gesammelte Werke Band 29: März – August 1919*, 5. Auflage (Dietz Verlag, 1953), 419; Vladimir Lenin, "A Great Beginning," *V. I. Lenin Collected Works, Volume 29, March-August 1919* (Progress Publishers, 1972), 429.
7 Mariarosa Dalla Costa and Selma James, *Die Macht der Frauen und der Umsturz der Gesellschaft* (Merve Verlag, 1973); Mariarosa Dalla Costa and Selma James, *The Power of Women and the Subversion of the Community* (Falling Wall Press, 1973).
8 Lise Vogel, "Hausarbeitsdebatte," in *Historisch-Kritisches Wörterbuch des Feminismus*, ed. Frigga Haug (Argument, 2003), 540–554, 544.
9 Vogel, "Hausarbeitsdebatte."
10 Anke Wolf-Graaf, *Frauenarbeit im Abseits. Frauenbewegung und weibliches Arbeitsvermögen* (Frauenoffensive, 1981), 220.
11 Peter Weiss, *Die Ästhetik des Widerstands* (Suhrkamp, 1975), 226; Peter Weiss, *The Aesthetics of Resistance*, trans. Joachim Neugroschel (Duke University Press, 2005), 199.
12 Virginia Woolf, *Drei Guineen*, trans. Anita Eichholz (Frauenoffensive, 1978), 46; Virgina Woolf, *The Three Guineas* (A Harvest Book, 1938), 81–82.
13 Karl Marx, *Das Kapital, Marx Engels Werke Band 23* (Berlin: Dietz, 1962), 381; Karl Marx, *Capital Volume 1, Marx and Engels Collected Works: Volume 35* (International Publishers, 1976), 365.
14 Karl Marx, *Das Kapital* III, *Marx Engels Werke Band 25*, 828; Karl Marx, *Capital, Volume III, Marx and Engels Collected Works: Volume* 37 (International Publishers, 1976), 807.
15 Editors' Note: The Hartz IV reform, introduced in Germany in 2005 as part of the broader Agenda 2010, represented a profound restructuring of the welfare and labour market system. Officially framed under the motto "Fördern und Fordern" ("Support and Demand"), the reform merged unemployment assistance and social welfare into a single benefit —*Arbeitslosengeld II* — and aimed to activate the unemployed through stricter obligations and sanctions. Critics, however, argue that Hartz IV marked a turning point toward neoliberal welfare policy. It reframed unemployment as an individual failure rather than a structural problem and placed recipients under constant scrutiny by Jobcenters. The system institutionalised precarious work, fostered the growth of the low-wage sector, and normalized insecurity as a permanent feature of life for millions. While unemployment figures declined statistically, this came largely through part-time and insecure employment.
16 Karl Marx and Friedrich Engels, "Die heilige Familie," *Marx Engels Werke Band 2* (Dietz, 1962), 3–224, 208; Karl Marx and Frederick Engels, "The Holy Family," *Marx*

and Engels Collected Works, Volume 4: Marx and Engels 1844–45 (International Publishers, 1976), 5–294.
17 Marx and Engels, "Die heilige Familie"; Marx and Engels, "The Holy Family."
18 Marx, Karl "Ökonomisch-philosophische Manuskripte," *Marx Engels Werke Band 40* (Dietz, 1968) 467–588, 535; Karl Marx, "Economic and Philosophic Manuscripts of 1844," *Marx and Engels Collected Works, Volume 3: Karl Marx March 1843-August 1844* (International Publishers, 1976), 229–346, 295.
19 *Mesa de Derechos y Cultura Indígena,* Grupo 4: *Situación, derechos y cultura de la mujer indígena*. See Frigga Haug, "Frauen von Chiapas," *Das Argument*, no. 217 (1996): 801–806.
20 Rosa Luxemburg, "Zur russischen Revolution," *Gesammelte Werke Band 4: August 1914 bis Januar 1919* (Dietz, 2003), 363; Rosa Luxemburg, "The Russian Revolution," *The Russian Revolution and Leninism or Marxism* (The University of Michigan Press, 1961), 78.
21 Bloch, *Tendenz – Latenz – Utopie*, 295.

References

Bloch, Ernst. *Tendenz – Latenz – Utopie.* Ergänzungsband zur Gesamtausgabe. Suhrkamp, 1978.

Costa, Mariarosa Dalla, and Selma James. *Die Macht der Frauen und der Umsturz der Gesellschaft.* Merve Verlag, 1973.

Costa, Mariarosa Dalla, and Selma James. *The Power of Women and the Subversion of the Community.* Falling Wall Press, 1973.

Engels, Friedrich. "Der Ursprung der Familie, des Privateigentums und des Staats." *Marx Engels Werke 21*. Dietz, 1962.

Engels, Frederick. "The Origin of the Family, Private Property and the State." In *Marx and Engels Collected Works, Volume 26*: *Engels 1882–89.* International Publishers, 1976.

Grimm, Jacob, and Wilhelm Grimm. *The Original Folk and Fairy Tales of the Brothers Grimm.* Translated and edited by Jack Zipes. Princeton University Press, 2014.

Haug, Frigga. "Frauen von Chiapas." *Das Argument*, no. 217 (1996): 801–806, citing *Mesa de Derechos y Cultura Indígena, Grupo 4: Situación, derechos y cultura de la mujer indígena* (febrero 1995).

Haug, Frigga. *Die Vier-in-einem-Perspektive: Politik von Frauen für eine neue Linke.* Argument-Verlag, 2008.

Lenin, Vladimir Iljitsch. *Gesammelte Werke, Band 29: März–August 1919*, 5. Auflage. Dietz Verlag, 1953.

Lenin, Vladimir Iljitsch. "A Great Beginning." In *V. I. Lenin Collected Works, Volume 29, March–August 1919.* Edited by George Hanna. Progress Publishers, 1972.

Luxemburg, Rosa. "The Russian Revolution." In *The Russian Revolution and Leninism or Marxism*. The University of Michigan Press, 1961.

Luxemburg, Rosa. "Die Proletarierin." In *Gesammelte Werke, Band 3: 3. Juli 1911 bis Juli 1914*. Edited by Annelies Laschitza and Günter Radczun. Dietz, 2002.

Luxemburg, Rosa. *Gesammelte Werke Band 4*: *August 1914 bis Januar 1919*. Dietz, 2003.

Luxemburg, Rosa. "The Proletarian Woman." In *The Rosa Luxemburg Reader*. Edited by Peter Hudis and Kevin B. Anderson. Monthly Review Press, 2004.

Marx, Karl. *Das Kapital. Marx Engels Werke 23*. Dietz, 1962.

Marx, Karl. *Das Kapital, Band III. Marx Engels Werke 25*. Dietz, 1964.

Marx, Karl. "Ökonomisch-philosophische Manuskripte aus dem Jahre 1844." *Marx Engels Werke Band 40*. Dietz, 1968.

Marx, Karl. "Capital, Volume 1." In *Marx and Engels Collected Works, Volume 35*. International Publishers, 1976a.

Marx, Karl. "Capital, Volume III." In *Marx and Engels Collected Works, Volume 37*. International Publishers, 1976b.

Marx, Karl. "Economic and Philosophic Manuscripts of 1844." In *Marx and Engels Collected Works, Volume 3: Karl Marx March 1843–August 1844*. International Publishers, 1976c.

Marx, Karl, and Friedrich Engels. "Die heilige Familie." In *Marx Engels Werke Band 2*. Dietz, 1962.

Marx, Karl, and Friedrich Engels. "The Holy Family." In *Marx and Engels Collected Works*, Volume 4: *Marx and Engels 1844–45*. International Publishers, 1976.

Vogel, Lise. "Hausarbeitsdebatte." In *Historisch-Kritisches Wörterbuch des Feminismus*. Edited by Frigga Haug. Argument, 2003.

Weiss, Peter. *Die Ästhetik des Widerstands*. Suhrkamp, 1975.

Weiss, Peter. *The Aesthetics of Resistance*. Translated by Joachim Neugroschel. Duke University Press, 2005.

Wolf-Graaf, Anke. *Frauenarbeit im Abseits. Frauenbewegung und weibliches Arbeitsvermögen*. Frauenoffensive, 1981.

Woolf, Virginia. *Drei Guineen*. Translated by Anita Eichholz. Frauenoffensive, 1978.

Woolf, Virginia. *The Three Guineas*. A Harvest Book, 1938.

Chapter 14

Interview with Frigga Haug[1]

Alexandra Colligs and Jeta Mulaj

Colligs & Mulaj: We want to start our conversation by talking about your famous essay "Victims or Agents" [*Opfer oder Täter*], which sparked considerable controversy and is currently translated in English as "Victims or Culprits?" How did this essay come about?

Haug: *Täter* is not culprits. Culprit—*culpa*—is not the correct translation and suggests that I am assigning guilt to women. The reason why this is important will become clear in a moment, when I describe the controversy following the essay.

As for how the essay came about, it is a bit of a funny story. The second women's movement, coming from the U.S., was spreading everywhere. I joined this movement as a student dropout, living in the countryside with a small child and a husband who was a student. Both of us had been members of the Socialist German Student Association [Sozialistischer Deutscher Studentenbund, SDS]. I had ended up in the country with a child and a husband, though all I really wanted to do was study forever. Studying was my goal and my practice. But, 12 semesters into the degree, everyone kept asking me when I would finally graduate. So, I had to do what others did—pick a topic and write a dissertation. I decided to write about *Subbotniks* in the Soviet Union, whom I imagined as a people who volunteered their labour, found it fulfilling, and wanted to change the whole society.[2] To do this, I first had to learn Russian. But, at the same time, I became pregnant and had a child. For women, a child is a trap. You love your child, but children are a trap that force you into a well-ordered life and well-ordered economy. Given the costs of raising a child, a middle-class job is necessary to bring home the money. Since women had fewer chances of getting a job—this was, you know, "everyday knowledge"—my husband got a job, and we moved near Cologne. I did not see the inside of the university for two years. I should have had the impulse to go to the university with the child, but somehow life with a child and studying don't mix well.

This trap of bourgeois life, as you can see, seemed to snap shut only for women. I really experienced what it meant to be a housewife. It's a life that makes one commit suicide, and yet you can't because of the baby. I despised being a housewife. I despised the women on the broadcast media where my husband worked, who were so cosmetic; they weren't my allies. I can't even say exactly why, but for me, they all seemed to have the wrong life. I became more and more unhappy, as the

DOI: 10.4324/9781003480143-14

people at the radio station became more and more cheerful. They were wrong, I was wrong, everything was absolutely wrong. I then said to this man I had the child with, in a calm voice, "By the way, I'm taking the child and I am moving back to Berlin to resume my life." He asked me when, and I said on Wednesday.

In Berlin, I went to the Action Council for the Liberation of Women. For the first time, I had a room full of women in front of me, all with long hair, talking, and it was there that I realized that I had spent my entire studies among men. Entering into this new life, my first transformative experience was to ally myself with women. Recognizing women as allies, as equal, and as different, but in any case, as a force, was essential for me. I soon realized that we needed a women's group. But the group that emerged, the Socialist Women's League of West Berlin [Sozialistischer Frauenbund Westberlin] quickly turned into women talking as mothers. I was still unhappy, but at least I was a bit rebelliously unhappy and decided to study the causes and origins of women's oppression; once we know that, I thought, we could rip it out by its roots. I turned the group into a training camp on women's oppression, history, and so on. Everyone studied. Women joined from all walks of life: librarians, secretaries, professors. From our studies came new questions: what do we do? How do we take action? We started organizing demonstrations, going into the public, and writing—really, developing into organic intellectuals. As we developed, more women started approaching us, describing their horrifying situations, stuck in abusive relationships with men who beat them. An outcry arose in me: *Why don't they fight back*? This was the main question that haunted me and eventually lead to the "Victims or Agents" essay. In part, I thought, they do not fight back because they produce their own oppression. Not alone, of course, but they produce it themselves. So, in part, I wanted to argue that women are not merely victims of their husbands, men, and some external social structures, but that they assist in creating their own oppression by following a historically necessary, or determined, path that leads them inside the home. But at once, it is precisely because it is in part women's own actions that contribute to this situation, they can change it!

I did think it was ludicrous for the Marxists to exclude me for making such an argument, which was already contained in Marx's "Theses on Feuerbach." I merely translated those theses into the politics of our time.

I wanted to challenge readers to consider how they themselves produce domination and contribute to their own subjugation through their participation in society. This perspective caused a scandal! It sparked controversy primarily due to a misunderstanding: some argued that I was attributing blame to women, suggesting they were guilty and at fault. But in truth, my intention was to investigate how women *participate* in society in ways that result in their oppression.

My thesis caused a scandal because it was interpreted in moral terms—as if I were saying "You are guilty or morally insane." I was seen as a traitor by most leftist groups and was eventually banished by the trade union, the German Communist Party [Deutsche Kommunistische Partei, DKP], and the left-wing Spartacus groups.

To this day, I am not sure why my essay provoked so much outrage. In a way, I thought I was saying what Marx had already said: people make their own history, but not under conditions of their choosing; people make history not out of their free will, but nonetheless they make it themselves.

Colligs & Mulaj: To understand the backlash you received, can you explain the relationship between the women's movement and the workers' movement at the time?

Haug: For many Marxists in parties and trade unions at the time, following *Capital* meant claiming that we must first liberate workers and only then would women become liberated. First, that is, we liberate workers from capitalism, and second, workers can liberate women, because they represent a second-order contradiction. So, the idea was that we must first deal with the main contradiction—between capital and labour—before we deal with women's liberation. Of course this is not what Marx claims, but nonetheless this position was adapted by those who opposed my essay. The workers also had their own personal aims, like having a housewife of their own, which made it easy for them to state that women shouldn't enter factory work, which is hellish. Instead, they claimed, women should stay at home and protect the children and make the house lovely and warm for their husbands—a stress-free, caring space. The factory is too awful for tender women; neither children nor women belong there.

Given this response, it is no wonder that the women's movement turned its back on Marx, and, in the worst-cases, treated all men as their enemies. The women's movement was not wrong in their observation that workers wanted women at home. And this historical animosity between the genders translated into the relationship between the two movements.

Colligs & Mulaj: How does the distinction between direct and abstract domination inform your analysis in "Victims or Agents"?

Haug: Direct domination is personal and overt, for example slavery, where you can see the enemy who is abusing and kneeling over you. By contrast, abstract domination—or, what I would also call veiled or structural domination—refers to how the entire society is organized; a domination that holds the whole world in disorder. The essay "Victims or Agents" explores both direct and abstract domination, arguing that women are complicit in their own domination, and that we can change the structures that we assist in creating in the first place.

The society in which we live has a particular form of domination such that any engagement in society represents both a way of being dominated and partaking in domination. Merely by being *in* society, one partakes in its mechanisms of domination. As a result, I wanted to redirect women's activity, strength, and anger from targeting men and structures in general toward recognizing their own activity in capitalist dynamics and domination. My claim was that the only way it is possible for you to change something in society is if you assisted in creating it in the first place. One must be an actor in the double sense—produce it and change it (or, at least intervene in it).

In this way, my essay was not primarily about whether domination in capitalism is direct or abstract, but *whose* activity it is. And, if it is *your* activity, then you have a part to play in being dominated and overcoming domination.

The direction of your question about domination raises questions about how to approach research aimed at liberation. When conducting research in universities, institutions, and neighborhoods, as I did, you encounter women who see themselves as "normal," that is, *not* dominated. To advance the goal of liberation, I found it necessary to form research groups together with the very people that the research is directly concerned with—workers, women, and the oppressed; even though, it is really difficult to do so.

Colligs & Mulaj: How did you address this difficulty? What was your approach to conducting research workshops with participants who had no background in theory?

Haug: For me, Marx's "Workers' Questionnaire" were immensely helpful. My research initially focused on whether automation increased oppression or offered greater opportunities for freedom and liberation. This question proved very challenging to answer, so I decided to visit automated chemical processing factories in Germany. At the beginning of our research, we wrote to a large number of companies asking about their degree of automation. This survey and its results were published in a first volume entitled *Automation in the Federal Republic of Germany* [*Automation in der Bundesrepublik Deutschland*] in 1975. This survey was necessary to counter the rumor that there was no automation worth mentioning in the Federal Republic of Germany. At the same time, it helped us to identify and write to the 64 companies where on-site investigations seemed worthwhile and actually took place. We soon published a volume on the development of work activities and the method for recording them. All these volumes are still available through *Argument* publishing house.

I wanted to talk to workers, but they were fixated in monitoring lights. The work of the control room attendant is invisible: he sits in front of a board where lights constantly flash. He observes whether dangerous deviations occur, whether everything is running according to its automatically controlled course. As he is a highly skilled worker, he knows how to read the signs he observes. We, however, stood outside and could not comprehend the activity we had come to observe. So, we didn't know what to ask. Eventually, one day, I mustered the courage and asked a worker directly: "What are you doing?" This departure from my usual inquiries about their activities, oppression, liberation—because as a Marxist, these were my ultimate concerns—startled him. He responded rather curtly in German, "Ich säuere" ("I sour") and then added, "Lights, lights." This response was both understandable for me and revealing, because it blended household language with abstract jargon. In this automated factory, there was a mix of very technical language and repetitive almost household-like activities. Workers spent all day monitoring and did nothing else; they watch all day, without much variation, occasionally pausing for coffee. This was their activity.

I studied around 60 such highly automated factories, where workers were not required to use their brains, ears, or touch. And yet something significant was happening with these workers that I wanted to capture. But, how could I capture it? Feeling desperate, I revisited Marx's "Workers' Questionnaire." Initially, I was almost disappointed by his seemingly mundane questions, like "How large is your workplace?" or "How far are you from the next worker?" These questions seemed too basic to reveal anything new. In fact, these questions seemed to be almost beneath the task of a researcher. But, as I wondered why Marx used these basic questions and what they might reveal, I realized the answer: Marx had changed their positions. He transformed workers into researchers of their own activity, workplace, and working conditions. Instead of merely being interviewed, the workers were led to investigate their own situation.

This powerful methodology turned the object of research into a researcher of their own situation in society and workplaces. Marx's questionnaire showed me that flipping traditional roles of subject and object empowers workers to analyze and critique their own activity and jobs. This was absolutely revolutionary. This realization struck me deeply, and I used a very similar approach to develop questionnaires for what became the victim-agent thesis. My aim was not just to document women's complaints about their real feelings of oppression, but to turn them into researchers of their own situation. Once you shift from being the object of research, you become the subject of research.

I embraced Marx's message: empower those you are researching to become subjects; transform everybody into researchers of their own lives and conditions, otherwise they cannot change anything. You can only change what you have assisted in constructing in the first place; or else, you are merely subject to domination, enslaved to a condition outside your control. But, since women are neither slaves nor passively dominated beings, the question for me became: how do women construct their own lives in such a way that they are not free?

I should note, the goal of this method is not about consciousness raising but transforming the questioner from a sufferer into an active researcher. It's a novel approach which I used with women, encouraging them not only to fight back but also to conduct research, to ask, where all of this comes from and how they can intervene more broadly in society. So, for me, the "Victims or Agents" essay was about initiating a different kind of women's research both within universities and, especially, in the workers' movement.

Colligs & Mulaj: So, as we have already discussed, your thesis in "Victims or Agents?" sparked quite an outrage. How was your broader attempt to connect feminism and Marxism received, especially with regard to the workers' and women's movements?

Haug: Many of my feminist interventions in Marxism were not initially well received. For example, my argument that gender relations *are* relations of production was considered a real offense to fighters of class struggle. Because the term "relations of production" is a holy term for class analysis, my saying that gender relations are relations of production was like stepping into church barefoot.

At the time, even participants at the International Marxist conference were primarily men. I remember attending one such conference in Yugoslavia with Wolf[3]—it was really important for our *Historical-Critical Dictionary of Marxism* to be surrounded by intellectuals from all over the world—only to find that there were just a few women. I believe only three, including myself and Donna Haraway.[4]

But, perhaps the most significant experience in this regard was my exclusion from Marxist and workers' groups. In 1980, I gave a lecture on the women's movement and socialism in a huge auditorium in the Free University of Berlin. This was historically significant because it marked a critical juncture between the workers' movement, women's movement, and socialism, and signaled the emergence of an open Marxist feminism. At the time, feminism was not regarded as honorable, and many Marxists dismissed it as an undesirable import from the U.S. Calling oneself a feminist, or even a female Marxist, was frowned upon. My lecture challenged the notion that socialism would come about solely through the workers' movement, which I criticized for its anti-feminist stance and its exclusion of women from its program. I argued that we needed a radical shift: women must be integral to socialism, which is a project about humanity, not men.

As a consequence of my position, I was excluded from Marxist groups, the Communist Party, the social democrats; none of them considered me a suitable member, resulting in my exclusion for four years. They even held a tribunal accusing me of hindering student activism and weakening their demands. Even my Doktorvater was against me, and another tribunal at the Marxist institute was held to confirm my expulsion. I was really shaken, but I thought to myself, "At least I have my students," only to find no one in the classroom. The Communist Party was very influential and had instructed students affiliated with it not to attend my seminars. So, my classes were empty, save for two or three so called "chaotic students."

Eventually, however, I was able to contribute to widening the idea of Marxism and to making it more dynamic, inclusive, and less dogmatic. I also co-founded the *European Forum of Socialist Feminists*, which included France, England, Italy, and Spain. I was able to do this because I was teaching abroad since, as a Marxist, I couldn't get a job in Germany for some time. So, I traveled country to country and brought socialist women together. The forum's main achievement was uniting and expanding the movement globally. To ensure longevity, we established a system where women served as advisors; each would begin as part of a group, but after a year, they would go on to start a new group. This cycle of mentorship and turnover helped sustain and grow the movement. All members were "on wheels"—not at home, but out there working to unite groups, students, and socialists. We even held a major congress in Frankfurt in 1972, where various socialist feminist groups met for the first time, and, where, for the first time, men were not allowed. It was also important that this was international because Germany at the time was not the right place, it was reactionary and had not recovered from fascism. The Forum was important in making Marxism less dogmatic. We met every two years in different countries where women sent their delegates. It is still going on today; last year it was held in Bilbao, Spain.

An important outcome was the "Thirteen Theses of Marxism-Feminism," which I formulated through collective processes and discussions during these Marxist feminist conferences. Conceived as a kind of manifesto, the idea is that all groups can discuss, revise, improve, and change the theses together. The theses are at once binding and open.

Colligs & Mulaj: We would like to return to something you mentioned earlier. You suggested that the workers' interests were aligned with confining women to the household. Could you explain what you mean by that a bit further?

Haug: I have done a lot of research with men in factories and found that many preferred traditional marriage: their wife at home with two kids, a boy and a girl, with the girl, of course, being slightly younger than the boy, and so on. However, these workers did not struggle to grasp that they were reproducing the oppressive structures in which women lived. In fact, it was much easier for them than for my students to admit the ways in which they are producing domination.

Colligs & Mulaj: This seems to be a typical bourgeois conception of the family, with the wife remaining at home and creating a sphere intended to counterbalance, what Marx and Engels in the "Communist Manifesto" describe as, the institutionalization of new social relations under capitalism, where people are connected only by naked self-interest—what they call the "icy water of egotistical calculation." What does this idea of the family mean for women?

Haug: One of the most insightful texts on the bourgeois family for me is Brecht's *The Seven Deadly Sins of the Petite Bourgeois*. It brilliantly explores the role of religion in constructing the bourgeois family through a ballet about a small family, who use their daughters' labour to secure their dream home—their private property. The story weaves religious justifications into the family's actions, which eventually even lead to turning their daughter into a sex worker. The only way in which the daughter can be a "good daughter" and not go astray—follow petty bourgeois rules—is, it turns out, by selling herself. The ballet has such fantastic lines, like "You have to do this out of love," to which the daughter responds by saying that women always love, but someone else, not the one with money. In all aspects, love becomes really awful, it becomes weaponized against women.

To return to your question, we are not dealing with a natural oppression of women simply because they have children and stay at home. Nor is this a heroic endeavor. We are dealing with women's oppression in capitalism. So, the question that consumed me was why must socialists engage in women's liberation if the main contradiction is that between capital and labour? This led me to study feminism, read authors like Sojourner Truth and Angela Davis, and ask: Why engage in women's liberation? Why form alliances with women, organize groups, and try to educate, rather than simply rely on capitalism or capitalist revolutionaries? These questions became more pressing as I realized that women faced oppression even within supposedly egalitarian student movements, like those in Russia and even Yugoslavia, which was, for a long time, the star on the horizon for us.

In the 1970s, a debate started within women's and socialist movements about domestic labour, why it is unpaid, and whether it should be paid. I felt that this approach missed the point; merely getting money in exchange for domestic labour would not solve any problems. It could merely expand wage labour and still keep domestic labour the domain of women. The debate was endless and very sophisticated, discussing percentages and proposing solutions for how women could juggle paid and unpaid labour. The latter being invisible and reproducing the wage worker who then provides for the family. The debates became tedious and overly technical but ultimately boiled down to the claim that part of women's labour is unpaid while men's is entirely paid, so we must fight over that percentage. It was all very boring to me—sophisticated and boring at the same time.

By thinking about this problem and living it—I was juggling writing and raising a child—I developed a different utopia, which I thought got us out of the circular debates around domestic labour that were still anchored in the form of our society. I called this new vision "a utopia by women for everyone." It was *by* women, because it took seriously reproductive labour and advocated for the need to fairly distribute it among all members of society, but it was intended for everyone. The starting point for this utopia was labour and time. We each have roughly 16 waking hours a day, outside of sleep and reproduction. Out of these, I allocated four hours to labour and another four to reproduction, four to self-development, and four to politics for everybody. Reproduction, it must be noted, was for everyone, not just for women. And self-development refers to activities one does to develop all sides of themselves, what Marx described as the fully developed individual, whether dancing or learning a new language. Thus, the utopia has a four-in-one structure.

Colligs & Mulaj: Can you say more about this reorientation of the social time regime within the Four-in-One perspective and how it came about?

Haug: The Four-in-One perspective emerged in response to the domestic labour debate, which I thought either devalued or romanticized reproductive labour. All of my reflections, whether Four-in-One or the analysis of women's oppression, start from the premise that we do not enter the world fully liberated, only to later be constrained by society, as if we step into a prison and then struggle to break free. Rather, domination is, in a sense, part of *you*—you act it out. The Four-in-One is meant to address these problems in a way that the solution focuses on balancing four areas: work, reproduction, self-development, and politics.

You can trace the development of this idea in everything I have written. It started with debates on domestic labour, where I was unsatisfied with the simple division of domestic versus wage labour. This led to a three-part perspective, which also proved insufficient, eventually evolving into the Four-in-One perspective as a response to the current division of labour and the domination of time. I thought the domestic labour debates were both one-sided and boring. I wanted to speak about the possibility of an emancipated society and not whether or not and how much exactly women contribute to surplus-value through this or that chore. The more sophisticated this theory became, the more boring it got—there was no emancipation, I thought, and no enthusiasm.

This was my intervention in the women's movement, the socialist movement, as well as in the workers' movement. It is indeed quite difficult to envision this four-sided development. Everyone is stuck in hierarchical and habitual ways of thinking, for example that "housework is bad," almost instinctively valuing it in this or that way. The Four-in-One perspective is meant more as a compass than a dogma where you simply follow a timer. Some of my students tried to implement it in this way with a clock and found that they could adjust it according to their immediate interests—they discovered that they don't need so much time in some activities and wanted to stress others more. Astonishingly, they increased labour time and got rid of the part where you take care of others, as a result, becoming like machines.

Colligs & Mulaj: So, they ended up prioritizing labour once more and reverting to the usual division of time?

Haug: Yes, precisely. Sometimes I worry that men might not like the Four-in-One perspective. I should ask Wolf if he likes it. I think he would, though he would prefer to get rid of housework entirely. He is good at it, but he might prefer not Four-in-One but instead working all day at his computer, writing critiques of Habermas—he would like a one-sided development. All time for work, 16 hours on Habermas. Don't you think this would be Wolf's utopia? Sixteen hours on Habermas?

Colligs & Mulaj: Sounds dreadful! But speaking of utopia, could you tell us more about how the Four-in-One Perspective relates to the possibility of a new society and to your vision of utopia?

Haug: I started exploring the idea of utopia out of curiosity about the ultimate goals of people's struggles. What do we want and what changes do women seek? As I was exploring this idea, my initial disdain was for the typical utopian vision of abundance, you know, streets filled with milk and honey, which seemed so boring and unappealing. It did not seem to represent what we actually want. Even in scenarios of scarcity and hunger, where the contrary is the case, and people are hungry and want to eat, we reach a stage where this is not enough, and we don't only want bread.

So, I kept asking: what is it that we want? Or, what is a possible account of what women also want? Having studied Marx, my first intuition was to include work in my vision of utopia, to avoid a condition where some people do not work because they subject others to work—you eat, while others work. Thus, work must be part of our vision of the future. Second, time was a crucial component since our active hours are limited. You need sleep, so you first put aside sleeping time—we do not want to do research in our dreams. So, how time is spent is important to consider. In the present, the majority of our time is spend working (more precisely, wage labour). In the utopia I envisioned, only a part of the 16-hour day would be devoted to work. Another part would focus on reproduction and a third part on self-development or learning new skills and developing oneself. It was really important for me to emphasize that everyone can engage in self-development, avoiding a scenario where one can learn 17 languages and how to play the violin, while others rot in labour; a condition where some learn a lot and others nothing. So, I wanted to incorporate Marx's idea of the fully developed individual. The fourth component is politics, or the organization of society. Everyone must engage in politics directly, not by means of representation, and take the organization of society into their own hands. So, my utopia was thus the Four-in-One perspective, represented by the image of a compass which contains the four sides. It was also a response to boring leftist slogans like one more euro per hour. I wanted to create another vision, located as a historical possibility, but that was new and compelling.

I first presented this vision of utopia to the Left in a beautiful, red, old Gothic mayor's house in Esslingen. Party representatives were invited to contribute to the idea, but they all lacked imagination—they could only think to ask for more money. I explained that the Four-in-One perspective was essential and that each element must be integrated and not left isolated; no one should be solely responsible for politics or the household. This revolutionary approach challenges our current division of labour or rather destroys it. Under this perspective, you cannot just be a housewife and care for your children because you need time to engage in politics and to develop yourself. Likewise, no one can just be a politician. Time must be allocated for all four aspects. When I presented this idea, no one opposed it but rather embraced it. It seemed perhaps more meaningful and less boring than fighting for an additional euro. If introduced in simple terms, this idea is understood by everybody as immediately relieving a burden from their shoulders— "I don't have to be a housewife; I don't have to be a politician."

This perspective represents a utopia for everyone, not just women. It is developed by looking at women but not solely concentrating on them. As I said earlier, I refer to this as building a utopia by women for everyone. It must be shaped by women because they will not overlook the reproductive aspect, even if they do so merely to rescue themselves.

Colligs & Mulaj: You mentioned that the Four-in-One perspective developed as a reaction to the debate on domestic labour and your dissatisfaction with tendencies to either glorify or devalue it. This reminds us of a line in your "Victims or Agents" essay about the possibility of breastfeeding becoming a pleasure. What did you mean by that remark, and what debates surrounded this topic at the time?

Haug: There was a heated discussion about breastfeeding in the women's movement. I did not want to negate the possible pleasure this activity could produce if it was not forced. But, I also wanted to insist that if such activities are *necessary* forms of labour, they cannot be sources of pleasure but only hard and compulsive work. In this way, I did not align with either position—those who condemned breastfeeding or those who adored it as a symbol of freedom and women's fulfillment. It seemed to me that the possibility of its pleasure could only be arrive at negatively.

So, as you can see, most of my arguments stem from contentious debates in movements, like this one. But, it was also informed by my experience. Unlike someone like my sister who loved breastfeeding, I had a difficult birth and was sick afterwards, so my baby was initially cared for by nurses. When I finally held her, breastfeeding felt very unfamiliar. Interestingly, it was my husband who purchased baby formula to avoid breastfeeding; he found it too corporeal and disgusting, and himself preferred the sterilized bottle. I never got used to breastfeeding—or this husband, who I got rid of. But, more importantly, I could not understand my sister who thought breastfeeding was a joy. To me, it was strange and painful. I never developed a relaxed relationship with it, so my experience was very different from the portrayal of it as a pleasurable, supernatural power.

Colligs & Mulaj: Let us now turn to another important aspect of your work: the feminist methodology developed under the title "Memory Work." Could you describe the process and the method?

Haug: Memory Work is related to Peter Weiss' claim that if we do not conquer liberation ourselves, it will have no impact on us. I always thought that this process begins with writing—from the head to the page. Writing about your condition is a fantastic start for women's epistemology.

The first thing that occurs when participants write down their memory—and it is on paper, in front of them, and they know they can rephrase it—is that they immediately start to rewrite it. Having it on paper allows them to intervene and say, "I did not mean it *that* way."

When we initially started the Memory Work groups, participants were allowed to rewrite their memory after we discussed it. But, to our surprise, the second version rarely added anything new. After the discussion, participants would often think, "Had I known this was important, I would have written it differently"; or, "You did not tell me in advance that this was important, so I must write it a second time." While this process was significant, and we even published a volume with these second versions, it made sessions endless.

Often, the rewriting wouldn't be very different, but sometimes the whole story changed. For example, after describing their oppression by the father in detail, they would want to rewrite everything to highlight that it was in fact the mother who was the source of the problem and who chased the father out. So, in a way, it may be a limitation of the method to allow rewriting several times—perhaps this does not necessarily lead us closer to the truth but further away from it. Even more, if you allow a second version to be written, why stop there? Why not a third, or fourth, or an infinite number of versions? Such processes may even make you lose interest in the person and her story, which is retold over and over again.

Another interesting thing that became evident during these sessions is that many women had a very impoverished vocabulary for expressing themselves and their miserable conditions. Often, they relied on just a few words like "do," "come," and "go"—their whole language treasure had just a few words that were endlessly repeated. Yet, the language they use was an alarm, an outcry. It highlighted their inability to express, and perhaps understand, their experiences beyond phrases like, "It is not in my hands," or "My situation is bad."

So, in many ways, Memory Work is work with language. You have only the material at hand (the written memory) and the author, who are one and the same. When language is limited, endless rewriting isn't helpful; even if the memory is rewritten a 1,000 times, it may reveal nothing. So, we needed to try something new to erupt out of these few meager expressions of their situation. For example, we created sheets with blank spaces for women to write down their activities, feelings or emotions, interests, and perspectives. When we looked at the results, much of the spaces were left blank—so many empty spaces.

What was striking was not just the empty spaces, but also that most women would not write answer any questions about their interests. They seemed to have no interests of their own. Even when they wrote about *themselves*, they had no interest. They didn't know them or couldn't find them...it was all very strange and sad. So, as always, we had to try to improve the method. To my reluctance, we eventually replaced "interests" with "wishes and hopes." This was done with the intention not to alienate women, but it also had the effect of making women appear as though they had wishes but no interests. Perhaps the association of the term "interest" with class made the term foreign to many. Interests seemed like something trade unions have, not us. Interests were seen as materialistic, you know, you shouldn't have interest but only wishes. As a woman you are so romantic—lots of wishes, but no interests. As if it is shameful to have naked interests. So, it turned out, it is easier to answer the question "what is your wish?" than "what is your interest?"

At every step, Memory Work as a method is also a language school—working with oneself and analyzing oneself in a Gramscian way. Women left "interests" blank because they had no language to express their interests. And our goal was not to inquire into their party affiliation or partner choices, but to see what language they use to describe themselves and their problems. It was, now I can see, naïve and silly to assume that everyone is able to speak about their interests.

Colligs & Mulaj: It is striking that, in Memory Work groups, the stories are written in the third person. Why did you make this choice, and how central is it to the overall methodology?

Haug: Yes, this was a deliberate choice. Writing in the third person helps avoid self-pity and increases accountability. The details become clearer and more precise. Then, in the group, we analyze the stories together and uncover all kinds of fascinating elements. Everyone becomes engaged, sees themselves as a storyteller, and also recognizes what is missing and why from the written account. A central question for us was always: what is being kept out? It is also essential that this work occurs in a group, which in a sense tests the plausibility of the stories. But, of course, this was a method and not a recipe, so we constantly changed and tried to improve it.

Colligs & Mulaj: One of the key themes developed in Memory Work is anxiety. Why did this particular theme become so central?

Haug: Yes, anxiety was the most developed theme in the workshop.

The goal of Memory Work was not to eventually fill in all the blanks on the sheet, but to seriously examine the given results; to scrutinize the empty spaces and to look at the written content collectively and in the open. This approach gives an impression of the person and the scene they are trying to portray, which often revealed themes of anxiety. We used this as a starting point to develop a theory of female anxiety. A far-reaching aim, but we began with the sentences in front of us.

When I first started the Memory Work, it was intended as a small, open seminar for women in the town, after I had been excluded from communist groups and workers unions. I wanted to focus on a theme that could engage ordinary women, not just university members and students. Based also on my own experience of walking home alone at night, anxiety seemed like an appropriate topic. To my surprise, the workshop was overcrowded.

In the stories and memories women wrote down during these workshops, female anxiety usually begins with depictions of oneself as alone in the world, without friends or anybody to rely on. This feeling of being alone makes nature appear closer, more dangerous, and threatening, with no possible option except flight. This was evident in how women depicted ordinary, little experiences. For example, a female worker from the suburbs of Stuttgart, where I live, in a recent session described her routine walk home, entitled "My Normal Way Home." What begins as an ordinary walk home becomes increasingly frightening. Anxiety starts to build and build, worsening when someone approaches and offers to accompany her; she declines, preferring to walk alone. Eventually, she goes down an underground path leading to the train platform, and the man follows her, making the situation worse and worse. As you read this story, you can easily experience it; it is familiar. It is composed of components of real danger for women in cities. You can easily sense the escalating danger for women in everyday settings like this.

Interestingly, the scene I wrote down when I started the workshop almost 40 years ago was almost identical to this one. Back then, missing the train meant having to cross a dark wooded area that felt like an abyss on the way home. It was so frightening to walk there, with men going in the same direction—ordinary men who seemed to acquire other characteristics as they walked into the dark abyss at midnight. So, I would typically call Wolf to come pick me up at the station instead. Similar scenarios of anxiety can happen in nature—the wind gets more intense, the storm grows louder, and the sounds of animals add to a growing sense of threat and danger for a woman alone.

These are all various expressions of anxiety. And we focused on anxiety, not *Furcht* [fear] which at least in German has a narrower and more directed connotation. Anxiety, however, is everywhere and requires no specific object.

The work we did with these stories full of anxiety was not intended as therapy but to provide women with a stable enough ground to navigate through the jungle of our society. It focuses on using language to describe and recognize oneself consciously. Ideally, it helps people manage their situations. That this process is collective is really important because it shows that these anxieties are not just fabricated but real ones shared by most women in the room.

When I was developing my account of female anxiety, there was a lot of tension in the Psychology Institute where I was teaching. The head of the institute, who had invented Critical Psychology, which was meant to be a Marxist psychology, was very suspicious of Memory Work. He thought it was ridiculous and unnecessary. As we began to view one another with suspicion, tensions in the institute arose—you know, I felt I was met with the look of "Who is this feminist coming here to mess up our wonderful, new, critical Marxist psychology?" While talking to him once—while I had my fear of walking alone at night in mind —I said, "Wait, let's imagine a scenario. A woman is walking alone at night through a dark park. It's getting darker. And all of a sudden she hears footsteps behind her...they approach faster and faster..." I didn't go on, the discussion stalled, and I couldn't get through to him. So, I tried a different angle: "Now imagine *you* are in the park, and this time, while walking, you hear the clicking sound of high heels following you. How do you feel?" He replied, "Oh, I would be pleased!" His reaction, and the laughter that followed, seemed to get the point across.

Anyway, in general, Memory Work, whether on anxiety or another topic, is challenging overall and presents a lot of resistances. Participants sometimes resist by saying that they don't want to change, "I am just as I am." Or, respond with indifference when asked about their wishes. For example, when asked why they like a certain thing in a certain way, they might say "I just do." If you ask them why they are afraid of the dark, they say "I just am." A resistance takes over, and they are reluctant to investigate and to alter their circumstances.

Colligs & Mulaj: In your work, you also write about daydreaming as a way of coping with and moving through seemingly hopeless situations—situations shaped by circumstances that appear beyond one's control. Can you explain why you claim that daydreaming can either replicate or reverse typical roles in existing society?

Haug: So many women daydream, almost as a habit. I started daydreaming when I found myself in the suburbs with a baby, while my husband went to work to earn money. With plenty of time on my hands, I spent hours dreaming of other things, imagining and inventing constellations. I did it so much that at some point I worried that I was going crazy, that this was a psychotic tendency in me or something awful. Curious, I asked women everywhere if they daydreamed; I even conducted surveys and found how common it is among women. I haven't come across men who daydream in the same way, though perhaps they do. I can ask Wolf, though I don't think he does; he's so focused and carefully separates his work from his free time.

I spoke extensively with women about their experience with daydreaming and was astonished by their responses—how it involves sitting, just being alive while being in another life at the same time. So many women shared similar experiences: "Oh, this one time, I was lost daydreaming and forgot the baby—It's out in the rain!" From the many stories I collected and analyzed, I was able to extract some the main traits and eventually publish on the topic. The volume of letters I received in response was overwhelming. I did not pursue this topic much further afterwards, as I somehow felt that the main features of it were visible, particular why one daydreams in certain situations when one feels unhappy but cannot feel unhappy. For example, when you have a baby, like I did, who demands your constant attention.

It is interesting that women's daydreams often reverse typical social roles. They position themselves as the lead, the one who is in control and can save their lover and loved ones from danger. This is a defining feature of daydreaming—you are the one, the lead, and *he* is entirely dependent on you. He will somehow die if you don't come to his rescue, like in the form of a cheap movie or a romance novel.

Colligs & Mulaj: Do you still daydream?

Haug: No, I have no time for it. Not only that, but I'm totally over-engaged in different projects all the time. But, I don't want to glorify or condemn daydreaming. You know, when I used to daydream a lot, I had a feeling that it wasn't, for a lack of a better word, normal. That I shouldn't do it; it felt almost like getting drunk, and I wanted to discipline myself. The more I analyzed and thought about it, I noticed a sort of need, especially from women, to compensate for something, to add something to their lives which are so poor. The accounts of women's daydreams are not fleeting moments; they are long elaborate scenarios.

But, I really do doubt that men daydream in this way, at least those who are fully devoted to the day's duties, who make life a duty. They turn life not into a dream but into a duty. For instance, when I am slowly waking up and jotting down little things here or there, Wolf's favorite saying to annoy me is: "You are wasting your day. Carpe diem." For him, it's *now*, only now. Now, you shouldn't hesitate. You can't dream and go to your world when you have so much to do. This is not exactly a question of the division of labour, as it is in the Four-in-One perspective, though it is a question about how to live and whether every bit of time should be filled with, say, writing. For example, in turn, I can annoy Wolf if I ask him funny questions or speak about trivial matters, like the new cat that arrived in our garden, during work time. We don't talk about cats when we work. So, this reaction pushes me to also turn to work immediately.

But, now I think of examples like *The Adventures of Tom Sawyer*, where Tom and his friend, Joe, take a long boat trip along the Mississippi River. Perhaps such fantasies, rather than daydreams, have a distinct gender character: they go into adventures, save women who are afraid, always encountering women in need of rescue, etc. Perhaps such visions are also manifest in daydreams—"When I grow up, I want to rescue a woman who will end up being my wife and the mother of my children."

You know, I once worked with a group of kids, between 10 and 15 years old, and asked them to write down one day in their future lives, the results of which are published in my *Frauen-Politiken.* What they described was both surprising and not surprising, because it was what you would expect of them if they were members of the capitalist society. It was awful and boring. Girls described finding rich husbands and having two kids. But, boys stepped out of the daily routine and became moon researchers, went into other worlds, and explored. Eventually, they returned home to their beautiful wife who was expecting them with chocolate pudding. But overall, it was a very dreadful repetition of everyday life culture, at least in Germany, and how boys and girls should be.

The different ways of living, not just daydreaming, between boys and girls that start so early on really interested me. I wanted to know when this gendered process starts. I found it very difficult to accept that the boys were much more interesting than the girls, who very early on stop asking and exploring and turn to look at the mirror instead.

When I discussed the results with the class, it was again the boys who were more interested in this process than the girls, who seemed less curious about the world. I have long given up on trying to provide a general theory for this gendering process especially because a lot of the women I work with do not represent such clichés.

Colligs & Mulaj: Staying with the theme of imagination, storytelling, and representation, we would now like to turn to literature, especially feminist detective stories, which have perhaps unexpectedly become an integral part of your work. Could you describe this project in general and explain how it connects to your more theoretical work?

Haug: Ah, *Ariadne*![5] The detective stories were such a success that we even managed to accumulate funds to pay for the translation of Gramsci's *Prison Notebooks* in German!

I found many insights about women's oppression in literature. For example, Christa Wolf's Büchner Prize speech is a fantastic summary of how women navigate oppression through the analogy of dance; step by step, dancing to the music, they are offered music of oppression, and Rossetta dances. She dances through the centuries, at one place she is burned, in another drowned, somewhere called Rossetta, elsewhere Marlene. Through dance—Dance, Rossetta, Dance—she conveys the fate of women across history.

But, to return to *Ariadne*. So, the women's movement was focused on a scientific study of women's oppression, its origins, and its possible overcoming. It was mostly without poetry. I, however, was a fanatic reader of literature, and I loved detective stories and crime stories. I only read them in private, though, embarrassed about reading such banal stuff in public. I read big books, you know, like *Capital,* and researched serious topics, and didn't waste my time with detective stories. So, I had to indulge on detective stories in private.

Then a publishing house in the U.K., called Women's Press, began publishing detective stories that I found very exciting. I read all of them alone, in silence, and in secret. I was so envious that they could publish such work, while I wrote about boring stuff, like women's oppression, domestic and wage labour. Eventually, I wondered, "Wait, why can't I do this too?"

To explore this possibility, I turned to the women's editorial board of *Das Argument*, established shortly after the journal's founding. Initially, as an editor, I found myself rejecting women's submissions because they did not meet the standards of this scientific Marxist journal. You had to be educated in Marxist theory to publish here; you couldn't just write about anything. As a result, women did not publish with us. Eventually, we decided that women must be part of the journal, and we promised to dedicate half of it to women's contributions. This proved to be an unattainable goal, since there were not that many women not just in the university but anywhere writing. As it was challenging to find enough qualified articles written by women on topics covered by the journal, we realized the need for an autonomous women's editorial board to intervene early in the topic selection process.

It was on this editorial board that I proposed creating a women's press to publish high-quality detective novels. Everyone, besides my daughter, opposed the idea. Together, she and I, and later other women who joined, launched an extra edition of feminist detective novels called *Ariadne*, named after the mythological figure who used a thread to navigate the labyrinth. The publication featured a range of feminist detective stories and was symbolized by the thread, connecting back to Ariadne's legend. This was enormously successful. I traveled all over the country, visiting various women's groups to discuss the project. I was surprised to find *Ariadne* crime novels everywhere, from kitchens and living rooms, to other countries, like Spain. In one village, where farmer women invited me to speak, I planned to talk about *Ariadne*, but to my surprise they all already knew of it. They wanted to discuss becoming poets and writers, engaging in politics, and changing the education of their children. They wanted to be researchers. They even brought up topics like homosexuality versus heterosexuality, which was a theme in some of the detective novels. One farmer even told me that she named her daughter after one of our lesbian heroines, E.R. Stoner McTavish, a name chosen to symbolize rebellion against oppressive friends and husbands.

Traveling and promoting the project was exhausting, but the effort paid off. We sold thousands of copies at a low price but still raised enough money to fund the translation of Gramsci's *Prison Notebooks.* It's strange, don't you think, that all this grew out of feminist detective stories?

Colligs & Mulaj: Indeed! *Das Argument*, which you just mentioned, has been an important part of your life and legacy. How did it come about, and what was your involvement in it?

Haug: At the time of atomic experiments in the Sahara and the German Army's consideration of atomic rearmament, a strong anti-atomic weapons movement emerged. We were actively involved in it, alongside a broad coalition—from leftist students to Christian churches, all united in a league for human rights. We organized sit-ins on the Kurfürstendamm, a famous avenue and shopping center in Berlin. We began with a group of 200 people sitting in the street protesting atomic weapons. We printed leaflets opposing the German Army's plan for atomic rearmament; a cause that should have been in everyone's mind after the horrors of Hiroshima and Nagasaki, but wasn't. We fought against the fact that it was easily forgotten.

In created leaflets offering to send additional information about our campaign against rearmament to anyone who sent us postage stamps. We called this initiative *Argument.* Günther Anders was amongst us as one of the founders.

At this time, I was about 28 years old and was less recognized than Wolf. My role initially was to collect material for issues. We worked out of Wolf's home, where we lived together; we had a floor to ourselves in an old, five-story house in Berlin with a storeroom in the attic. It was very cheap, with many stairs and no elevator. I recall how challenging it was to climb to the fifth floor with a baby on my hip.

Initially, before I moved in with Wolf, he was in Italy and France learning languages, and I was married to the father of my baby. I still had to finish my dissertation, but I misunderstood the necessities of caring for a baby. As I mentioned earlier, they sort of consume all your time, at least in the beginning. They consume your life. Even if they are well and happy, they consume your life and interests; everything revolves around the baby. When Wolf returned to Berlin, he complained that I was always talking about the baby and what the baby needs. It was difficult to come back to a life of research instead of looking at the smiling baby.

When the child was about two years old, I put her in one of those backpacks from which they can look out and returned to the university with her. By then, *Das Argument* was already in leaflets, having begun as an anti-atomic movement. The baby was born in 1963, and the anti-atomic movement started in the 50s, so, unlike the baby, it was already over ten years old. The baby did not stop my work; though that situation was difficult to navigate, it connected me to everyday life and its management in a way that eventually led me to develop the Four-in-One perspective.

Notes

1 This interview, which was conducted in both English and German, took place in Frigga Haug's residence in La Palma in the span of three days, from January 13th to 16th of 2023.

2 Editors' Note: *Subbotniks* refers to days of unpaid, voluntary community labour in the USSR. Although it began as a spontaneous grassroots movement during the Russian Civil War, it was later institutionalized and imposed by the Soviet government.

3 Editors' Note: Frigga is here referring to her husband, Wolfgang Fritz Haug, who she calls by the nickname "Wolf."

4 Editors' Note: Frigga is here referring to the *Historical-Critical Dictionary of Marxism*, which is a multi-volume Marxist encyclopedia.

5 Editors' Note: Established in 1988, *Ariadne*, founded by Frigga Haug, is the political crime fiction series published by Argument Verlag. Dedicated to feminist crime literature, the series featuring both translations of international women authors and works by German-language writers.

Index

Note: Page numbers followed by 'n' refer to notes.

For Product Safety Concerns and Information please contact our EU
representative GPSR@taylorandfrancis.com
Taylor & Francis Verlag GmbH, Kaufingerstraße 24, 80331 München, Germany

www.ingramcontent.com/pod-product-compliance
Ingram Content Group UK Ltd.
Pitfield, Milton Keynes, MK11 3LW, UK
UKHW020008200926
475702UK00015B/2538

* 9 7 8 1 0 3 2 7 6 8 0 1 4 *